ཀུན་མཁྱེན་རྫོང་ཆེན།

PATH TO RAINBOW BODY

Introduction to Yuthok Nyingthig

Dr. Nida Chenagtsang

Copyright © 2014 Dr. Nida Chenagtsang སྨན་པ་ཉི་ཟླ་ཚེ་དབང་།

Published by Sorig Press

2014 Edition
Printed in the United Kingdom
Cover Design Copyright © Sorig Press

All rights reserved. No part of this book maybe reproduced without prior written permission from the Publisher or the International Academy for Traditional Tibetan Medicine.

ISBN 978-1-909738-09-6

A special mention of gratitude to all those whose valuable contributions made this work possible.

Contents

Preface	IX
Foreword by Robert A. F. Thurman	XI
Editor's Introduction to the New Edition	XIII

YUTHOK NYINGTHIG ROOT TEXT	**3**
Ngöndro	7
Common Ngöndro	8
Uncommon Ngöndro	9
Routine Ngöndro	10
Kyerim	12
Outer Guru Yoga	13
Inner Guru Yoga	14
Secret Guru Yoga	14
Concise Guru Yoga	14
Dakini Practice	15
Dzogrim	16
Tummo	18
Dream Yoga	19
Clear Light Yoga	19
Illusory Body Yoga	20
Bardo Yoga	20
Phowa	21
Karmamudra	22
Mahamudra	24

Dzogchen	27
Additional Practices	30
Eliminating Obstacles	30
Signs of Practice	31
Medical Action Practice	31
Long Life Practice	32
Fire Puja	32
Amulet	33
Pulse Practice	33
Protector Practice	33
COMMENTARIES	**35**
Zurkhar Nyamnyi Dorje	36
His Holiness the 5th Dalai Lama	37
Kongtrul Yönten Gyatso	38
Karma Jigme Chökyi Senge	39
HISTORY OF YUTHOK NYINGTHIG	**41**
Yuthok the Elder (729 - 854)	42
Yuthok the Younger (1126 - 1202)	45
Yuthok's Song	48
Yuthok Nyingthig Lineage	55
APPENDICES	**59**
List of Yuthok Nyingthig Contents	60
Explanations on Vajrayana	66
Origin of Tibetan Buddhism	66

Major Schools of Tibetan Buddhism	67
Chöd	68
Rime	69
Vajrayana System	69
Vajra Body	74
The Guru	76
Transmission System	77
Samayas	82
Base, Path and Result	84
Glossary	87
Bibliography	103
Index	105

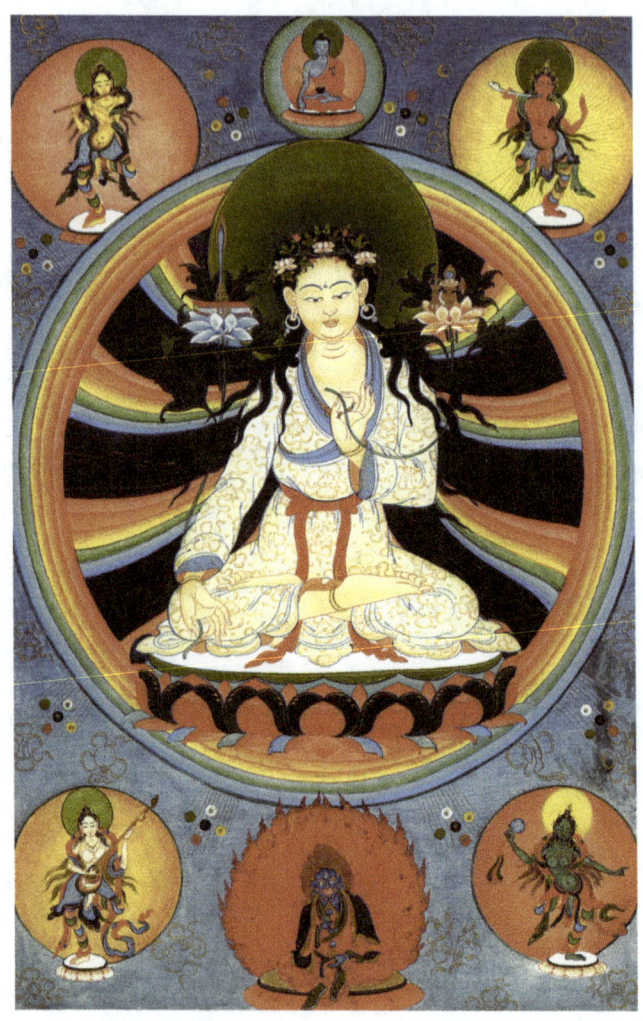

Yuthok and the Four Dakinis, with Medicine Buddha above and Shanglon below

VIII

Preface

Path of Rainbow Body
Yuthok Nyingthig is the most important spiritual practice for physicians and healing practitioners of Traditional Tibetan Medicine. Yuthok Nyingthig means 'The Innermost Essence of the Teaching of Yuthok'.

This practice was composed with the intention of imparting a profound and harmonious understanding to doctors, health and allied health care specialists alongside dharma practitioners, giving them the opportunity to experience the union of medical practice and spiritual practice. This perception is realized in the most essential and subtle form of the five elements through body, mind and energy.

The Yuthok Nyingthig practice brings about spiritual progress, good health and longevity for all those who practice it. I should also emphasize that it enhances diagnostic and therapeutic abilities for physicians. These aspects of the practice are considered the relative goal.

While the goal of the Yuthok Nyingthig practice is geared towards a spiritual growth, whereby the practitioner attains a deeper level of perception and experience on the way to spiritual awakening, the ultimate goal is treading the spiritual path that leads to the Rainbow Body, the highest aspect of spiritual realization.

Based on the great Yuthokpa, the King of Medicine's promise, I think that when one is a medical practitioner who follows in his footsteps, it is extremely important to exert oneself in practicing this Nyingthig Guru Sadhana for seven days at the very least, or as a daily practice. Consequently, I hope that the publishing of this edition will be of great benefit to the physicians of today, regardless of whether they are familiar with this Dharma Cycle or not.

Dr. Nida Chenagtsang
Medical Director
International Academy
for Traditional Tibetan Medicine
May 2014

Foreword

Dr. Nida's Path to Rainbow Body provides a wonderful, initial overview of the marvelous teaching of the Yuthok Heart Essence, the principal spiritual teaching employed in Tibet for the training of physicians in continuous use in Tibetan medical schools since the 12th century, the time of Yuthok Yönten Gönpo the Younger. I first encountered this amazing work and practice when I briefly studied Tibetan medicine at the Tibetan Medical and Astrological Institute in Dharamsala, India under the Master Doctor Yeshi Dhonden in 1964-5. I am delighted that Dr. Nida is carrying on this precious tradition so deeply and expansively in Tibet, Asia, and the West, healing patients, teaching physicians, and publishing numerous books and articles such as this clear and authentic summary.

The famous Gyud Shi, or Four Tantras, are the exhaustive textbooks the Tibetan doctor must master, covering every aspect of life and sickness and healing of mind and body. Complementarily, the Yuthok Heart Essence remains the essential educational curriculum of contemplative cultivation of the doctor's own mind and spirit, enabling her or him to develop wisdom, replete with the intuitive clairvoyant insight into the condition of patients' bodies and minds that enables the doctor to be a competent healer, and the open-hearted compassion for the suffering patients that inspires the doctor to become one. It is taught that one should not take up the vocation of doctor if motivated by desire for wealth, fame, or status - one must be motivated by unswerving compassion. If one is sincerely so motivated, however, success in lesser worldly aims is assured, as patients who have received true benefit will inevitably be grateful. Therefore, the first, not the last, aspect of a doctor's education is in the method of cultivating such a true compassion.

This small book gives a brief but thorough introduction to this unique method of the doctor's essential inner training that must precede and complement the vast external learning that must be mastered over many years of medical school and early practice. It is my privilege and pleasure to add my enthusiastic recommendation of the excellence of Dr. Nida's work.

Robert A. F. Thurman
Jey Tsong Khapa Professor
of Indo-Tibetan Buddhist Studies,
Columbia University
President, Tibet House U.S.
May 2014

Editor's Introduction to the New Edition

The Yuthok Nyingthig Root Text is an exposé of Yuthok's spiritual teachings. It was composed in the twelfth century as part of what was later to be known as 'The Two Jewels' by Yuthok the Younger.

'Gyud Shi', the Four Tantras, was how this text was originally named and it refers to the relative aspect of Sowa Rigpa, the 'Science of Healing', a native term for Traditional Tibetan Medicine. It is the most basic and standard reference text for any physician or practitioner of Tibetan Medicine. The Yuthok Nyingthig, regarded as the second jewel, refers to the absolute aspect of Sowa Rigpa, which, in this case is translated as 'Nourishment of Awareness'.

Yuthok considered spiritual practices, yoga and meditation to be an integral part of every physician's training, and, in fact also of non-medical practitioners, especially the busy and the lazy. The Yuthok Nyingthig practice itself is associated with the development of special powers of omniscience and clairvoyance which aid the physician in becoming a greater healer.

Dr. Nida Chenagtsang received the transmission of the Yuthok Nyingthig from Khanpo Toru Tsenam and Khonpo Tsultrim Gyaltsen, and, in turn is committed to the transmission of this great spiritual practice. Both students of Tibetan medicine as well as students or practitioners of other medical and healing practices who show sincere dedication to the healing tradition of Tibetan medicine may receive this transmission.

This 'Introduction to Yuthok Nyingthig' was written in order to give an overview of Yuthok's complete Dharma Cycle to both new and experienced practitioners of the Yuthok Nyingthig.

In this new edition, the title 'Path of Rainbow Body' was changed to 'Path to Rainbow Body', along with some corrections and new information added by Dr. Nida Chenagtsang.

The books publication date in June 2014 mirrors Yuthok's transmission of his complete teachings to his heart disciple Sumtön 800 years ago in the Monkey Month of the Horse Year. May it be as auspicious!

Tam Nguyen, MD
Editor
International Academy
for Traditional Tibetan Medicine
May 2014

"If the supreme teaching of the Guru Sadhana Dharma Cycle of the Yuthok Nyingthig did not have the blessing of simultaneous practice and accomplishment, then the people of the degenerate age, entangled in worldly desire and weak in determination for long retreats, would not be able to practice.

However, if this, the accomplishment of my life-force itself, is practiced without distraction by a faithful person for seven days, then I vow that I shall reveal well my face to them, and I shall grant them teachings and closely instruct them."

Yuthok Yönten Gönpo, 12th century

གཡུ་ཐོག་སྙིང་ཐིག་གི་རྩ་བའི་སྐོར།

YUTHOK NYINGTHIG ROOT TEXT

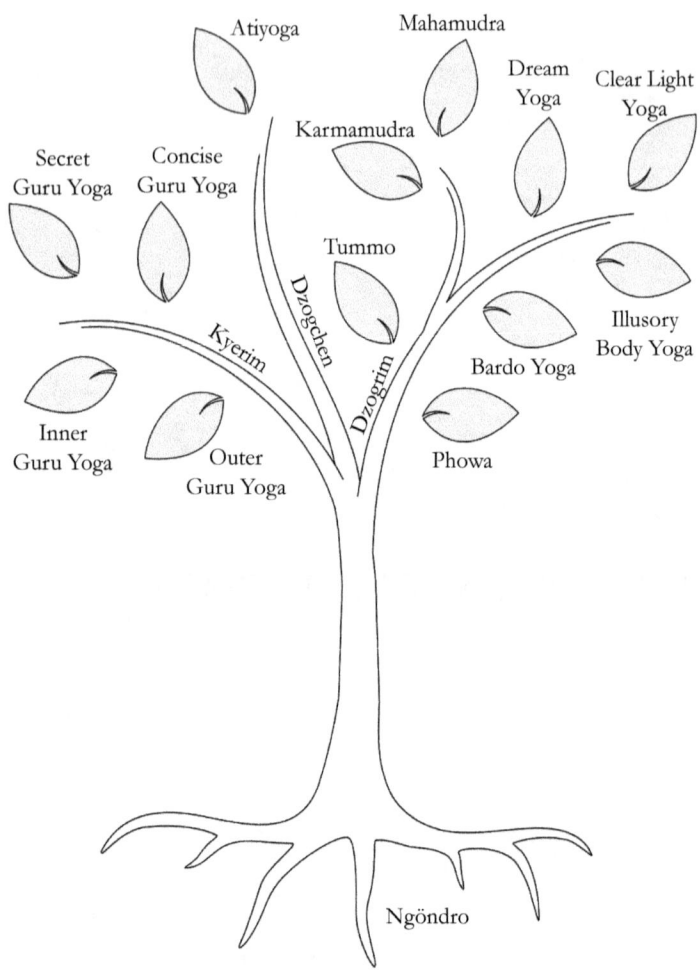

'Yuthok Nyingthig Tree', a schematic depiction following the creative educational tradition of Sowa Rigpa

The root text of Yuthok Nyingthig can be categorized into following divisions and subdivisions:
1. Ngöndro (Preliminary Practice)
   a. Common Ngöndro
   b. Uncommon Ngöndro
   c. Routine Ngöndro
2. Kyerim (Creation Stage)
   a. Outer Guru Yoga
   b. Inner Guru Yoga
   c. Secret Guru Yoga
   d. Concise Guru Yoga
   e. Dakini Practice
3. Dzogrim (Completion Stage)
   a. Tummo (Fire Yoga)
   b. Dream Yoga
   c. Clear Light Yoga
   d. Illusory Body Yoga
   e. Bardo Yoga (Transitional State Yoga)
   f. Phowa (Transference Yoga)
   g. Karmamudra (Action Seal)
   h. Mahamudra (Great Seal)
4. Dzogchen (Great Perfection)
5. Additional Practices
   a. Eliminating Obstacles (Eliminating Secret Obstacles)
   b. Signs of Practice (Eliminating Inner Obstacles)

c. Medical Action Practice (Eliminating Outer Obstacles)
d. Long Life Practice
e. Fire Puja (Offering Ritual)
f. Amulet
g. Pulse Practice
h. Protector Practice

Ngöndro

Common Ngöndro	8
Uncommon Ngöndro	9
Routine Ngöndro	10

Ngöndro (Tibetan: སྔོན་འགྲོ, *Wylie: sngon 'gro*) means preliminary practice or preparation. The term 'preliminary' refers to something very basic yet very profound and of great importance - an essential basic practice, a tree's roots. As with the upbringing of a child, where family and early school education are both rudimentary yet important aspects of the child's development, in a similar way, the Yuthok Nyingthig Ngöndro practice is both essential and extremely useful for beginners as a means of envisioning the value of life and making progress in the spiritual practice.

Another metaphor would be the building of a house. As the foundation needs to be very strong to later build more sophisticated floors and structures upon it, likewise, the development of spiritual practice needs a stable basic framework. The historical Buddha mentioned ten bhumis, literally meaning grounds or levels, of a Bodhisattva's spiritual development until reaching full enlightenment.

In the Tibetan Buddhist tradition, Ngöndro practices are often very demanding with regards to time and effort. Strong dedication is needed to accomplish at least 100,000 prostrations, 100,000 recitations of refuge and bodhicitta, 100,000 Mandala offering, etc. However, the Yuthok Nyingthig (Uncommon) Ngöndro takes only seven days, thus sustaining Yuthok's special blessing as to speed.

Typically, in other Ngöndro practices there are two different stages referred to as Common Ngöndro and Uncommon Ngöndro, but the Yuthok Nyingthig Ngöndro is made up of three main parts: Common Ngöndro, Uncommon Ngöndro and Routine Ngöndro.

Common Ngöndro

The Common Ngöndro is known as 'Four-Fold Mind-Changing'. It is the foundation of further specific practices and is called Yuthok Nyingthig Ngöndro in the root text. It is called Common Ngöndro because it is generally meant for any kind of spiritual practitioner and leads one to reflect upon the meaning of life and see its true value.

The four thoughts our mind should focus on and change its attitude toward are:
- The difficulty in achieving a precious human life
- The impermanence of life

- The natural law of cause and effect
- The consequence of living in Samsara.

This will lead to
- The benefits of spiritual liberation.

Uncommon Ngöndro

This is a special Buddhist concept which differs from the usual way of looking at life. Dharma in general refers to a way or path, and everybody and every tradition has their own way of thinking and living. The Buddha's view is called Buddha Dharma which in the Buddhist tradition is called Uncommon (to others). In the Yuthok Nyingthig tradition, there are seven main aspects of it:

1. Refuge (protection by the Three Jewels)[1]
2. Bodhicitta and the Four Immeasurables (training of mind in loving kindness)
3. Prostration (body purification)
4. Mandala offering (practicing generosity)
5. Circumambulation (mindful walking meditation)
6. Dorje Sempa practice (purification of negative karma)
7. Kusali practice (reduction of attachment and fear)

---

[1] The traditional way of treating the disease of Samsara is to view Buddha as the physician, Dharma as medicine, and the Sangha as nurses.

Routine Ngöndro

Once the Uncommon Ngöndro is completed, a routine practice needs to be established. Importantly, this is something that can be practiced throughout one's entire life, whenever practitioners can or desire to do something for the benefit of others, to help others and make others healthy and happy. This routine practice can also be called Karma Yoga.

By integrating daily life into the practice, it ensures mindfulness in every aspect and in every action of life. In the original text there are six important points:

1. Be involved in charity projects especially those that help the poor and the sick.
2. Find ways to save the lives of people and animals.
3. Always strive to spread Buddha's and Yuthok's teachings, especially the Four Medical Tantras and the Yuthok Nyingthig.
4. Create a clinic or a centre where those who are in need can receive help.
5. Make donations or offer your time to help build things that will benefit many beings[1].
6. Take care of abandoned animals[2] and protect the environment[3].

---

[1] such as community centers, animal shelters or wells and bridges in poorer countries
[2] by feeding them, giving them medical treatment and saving their lives
[3] by reducing, recycling and reusing materials

This reflects in the Buddha's simple words "Strive for good deeds as much as possible, avoid negative actions as much as possible, and tame your mind. This is the Buddhist tradition."

The union of compassion and wisdom in all aspects is essential. It means having smart love and skillful kindness. Conditioned or blind compassion, on the other hand, can lead to further problems and conflict, such as giving money to people with addictions who will only buy more harmful substances for themselves, or liberating animals into a habitat where they cannot survive. These examples show the importance of a wise view regarding long-term consequences in order to truly benefit sentient beings.

Kyerim

Outer Guru Yoga	13
Inner Guru Yoga	14
Secret Guru Yoga	14
Concise Guru Yoga	14
Dakini Practice	15

Complementary to the basic Buddhist refuge in the Three Jewels, Buddha, Dharma and Sangha, Vajrayana Buddhism introduces refuge in the Three Roots, Guru, Deva, Dakini, which can be found in the Yuthok Nyingthig Kyerim practice. As opposed to the Outer Tantras, where one visualizes the deity as separate from oneself, Kyerim usually engages in visualizing oneself as the deity (Tib. Yidam). It is therefore also known as 'Deity Yoga'. The goal is to transform ordinary conception and perception by creating a divine self, increased positive pride and stable mental clarity.

Vajrayana's Kyerim is the equivalent of the Sutrayana Samatha.

The Yuthok Nyingthig Kyerim creation stage, is presented through four forms of Guru Yoga where Yuthok is guru, under various appearances of different Buddhas or Devas, and via two dakini practices that follow. The Yuthok Nyingthig practice is an all in one practice of Guru Yoga where Yuthok Nyingthig takes on the form of Guru, Deva and Dakini. As part of the Mahayoga, it marks the first stage of meditative practice of the Inner Tantras, complemented with the completion stage (Anuyoga) from these.

According to Yuthok's teaching, Guru Yoga is the absolute key point to eliminating and transforming all destructive emotions or obstacles, and to discovering our innermost transcendental wisdom or pure pristine awareness. Through this extraordinary blessing, there is hope in achieving instant realization.

Outer Guru Yoga

The Outer Guru Yoga focuses on Yuthok with the Four Medicine Dakinis. It includes the Four Empowerments and the mantra of the entire Outer Yuthok Mandala. The Yuthok Guru mantra is introduced in the Inner Mandala. The Outer Guru Yoga can be summarized as meditation on the guru as a refuge field.

The whole practice is compressed into a seven day retreat. It is followed by the practice of Four Activities including a meditative healing practice which is unique to Yuthok Nyingthig.

Inner Guru Yoga

The Inner Guru Yoga includes Kyerim and Dzogrim. The Kyerim practice focuses on Yuthok in the form of Medicine Buddha and includes the practice of the Five Buddhas opening the five chakras. The Dzogrim practice is about Clear Light. Altogether, this meditation on the guru as Buddha is a seven day practice. Additionally there is a meditative study of the Four Tantras.

Secret Guru Yoga

This practice is a meditation on the guru as union of the Three Roots. The self visualization is the union of Hayagriva and Vajravarahi. This practice also works with the channels and chakras and combines Kyerim and Dzogrim in seven or more days of practice. There are two practice versions of the Secret Guru Yoga: a simplified one and a more elaborate one.

Concise Guru Yoga

In the Concise Guru Yoga, Yuthok appears in the form of Vajrasattva in union with his consort. This practice is termed concise due to its simplification. It is a daily guru yoga practice and includes a long life practice.

Dakini Practice

To complete the practice on the Three Roots, the Yuthok Nyingthig contains special dakini practices which follow the guru yogas.

Dzogrim

Tummo	18
Dream Yoga	19
Clear Light Yoga	19
Illusory Body Yoga	20
Bardo Yoga	20
Phowa	21

The next stage of practice called Dzogrim or 'Completion Stage' consists of the Six Yogas of Naropa which are very well known in Tibet. They include Tummo, Illusory Body, Clear Light, Dream Yoga, Bardo and Phowa. The Six Yogas of Niguma are almost identical to the Six Yogas of Naropa and only differ in that they are taught by the female master Niguma.

Since the 11th century, the Six Yogas are mostly practiced in the Kagyu and Nyingma schools. They are mentioned as the practice of Anuyoga, but the Gelugpa's five stages of practice are also very similar, including silence of body (illusory body), silence of voice, silence of mind, clear light and union. The terminology differs, however the method of practice remains essentially same.

The Six Yogas are an advanced chain of practices from Anuttara yoga tantra; it is the main body of completion stage practice. Profound knowledge of the subtle structures of the Three Vajras is necessary in order to fully understand and realize the Six Yogas. The main goal is to achieve the blissful and clear light natured state of Buddhahood. This happens through the discovery of one's own infinite potential and through realizing the true nature of the vajra body, vajra speech and vajra mind.

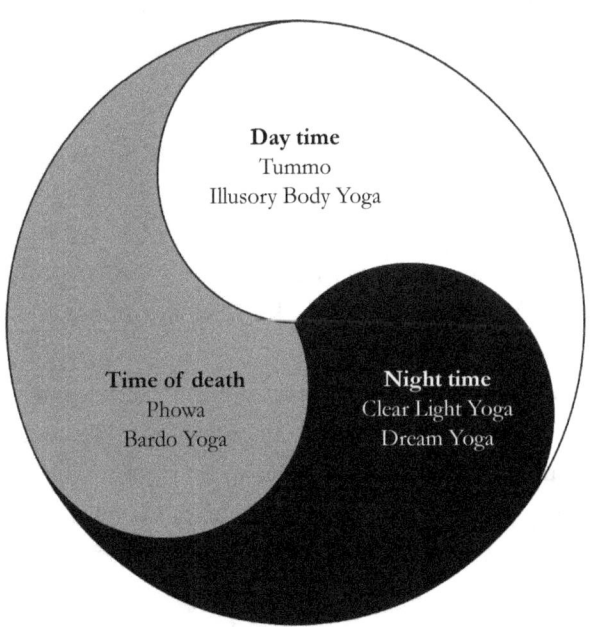

In the Yuthok Nyingthig Root Text the practices of the Six Yogas are introduced in the 19th chapter 'The Self-Arising Three Kayas of the Completion Stage'. There is no timeframe mentioned for any of the yogas but it is said that each one is practiced in a retreat "until it is completed".

The Six Yogas are the practice of the cycle of life and death and some are to be practiced during the day or at night time, depending on which cycle they correspond to. Tummo and Illusory Body Yoga are to be practiced during the day as they correspond to the life cycle. Clear Light Yoga and Dream Yoga belong with the death cycle and are to be practiced at night and Phowa and Bardo are to be practiced at the time of death.

Tummo

The complete name of Tummo is གཏུམ་མོ་བདེ་དྲོད་རང་འབར། *(gtum mo bde drod rang 'bar)* The Divine Fire Yoga of the Self-Blazing Blissful Heat.

Tummo is the foundation of other practices including Karmamudra. It purifies all negative energies and bad karma and enhances innate bliss and wisdom. It is a practice that generates the inner divine fire element to eliminate the root of all imbalance and increase perfect bliss and wisdom.

Tummo is complemented by a dark retreat of 7 days and the practice of Bumbachen.

Dream Yoga

The complete name of Dream Yoga is རྨི་ལམ་ཉིད་འཁྲུལ་རང་དག *(rmi lam nying 'khrul rang dag)* The Dream Yoga of Self-Purified Illusion.

Dreaming is the middle state between the waking state and the state of death, hence dream yoga is a bridge between life and death. It is also known as the check point, because a good dream yoga practitioner has no worries about the bardo. By practicing dream yoga one achieves the hidden activity of mind and energy, freeing oneself from all types of blockages and troublesome emotions.

Clear Light Yoga

The complete name of Clear Light Yoga is འོད་གསལ་གཏི་མུག་རང་སངས། *('od gsal gti mug rang sngas)* The Clear Light of Self-Awakened Ignorance.

Clear Light is the most essential aspect of the Six Yogas. Through it, the great illusion of samsara will be removed and the true nature of mind and awareness of presence is understood. Child Clear Light is the clear light experience that a practitioner can achieve and it is in preparation for the process of death. During the death process, the innate Mother clear light can be realized. The 'Union of Mother and Child Clear Light' is the terminology used when one dissolves in that light and this is known as spiritual realization.

Illusory Body Yoga

The complete name of Illusory Body Yoga is སྒྱུ་ལུས་ ཆགས་སྡང་རང་གྲོལ། *(sgyu lus chags sdang rang grol)* The Illusory Body of Self-Liberated Attachment And Aversion.

Illusory body is an essential support for Tummo, and it helps the mind to be free from attachment and aversion and to discover and experience the real nature of the body and all existence. The eight similes of illusions commonly used by practitioners are: dream, magic, hallucination, mirage, echo, town of spirits, reflection, apparition.

Bardo Yoga

The complete name of Bardo Yoga is བར་དོ་ལོངས་སྐྱུ་རང་ འཆར། *(bar do longs skyu rang shar)* The Intermediate State of the Self-Manifested Sambhogakaya.

Bardo is a method of preparation for obtaining a pure illusory Sambogakaya, in other words, enabling the practitioner to make a choice for the next rebirth. It familiarizes the practitioner with the process of dying which, in turn, leads to total freedom after death.

Phowa

The complete name of Phowa is འཕོ་བ་མ་སྒོམ་སངས་རྒྱས། *('pho ba ma sgom sngas rgyas)* The Transference of Consciousness As Liberation Without Meditation.

Phowa is considered a shortcut to enlightenment. It is like a first aid for the practitioner to be ready for the time of death. It is considered a practice on how to die in peace for the final spiritual journey to the pure land of the Medicine Buddha.

Dzogrim

Karmamudra

Karmamudra is the practice of the orgasm state which is naturally experience in the head and base chakra. 'Karma' means action, 'mudra' means gesture or partner, together Karmamudra is known as the 'path of bliss' or the 'union practice'. This practice can be done alone or with a partner, and it is suitable for young and active people.

There are two aspects of the practice, རང་ལུས་ཐབས་ལྡན། *(rang lus thabs ldan)* self practice and the གཞན་ལུས་ཐབས་ལྡན། *(gzhan lus thabs ldan)* practice with a partner.

Through maintaining awareness during the practice one can understand the nature of mind. It also involves training in yogic exercises and utilizing the energy and channels to attain different levels of bliss experiences to integrate with meditation, for both men and women.

The nature of emptiness can be understood through the experiences of the དགའ་བ་བཞི། *(dga' ba bzhi)* Four Blisses and the སྟོང་པ་བཞི། *(stong pa bzhi)* Four Emptinesses. They are obtained through the practices of Tummo and Karmamudra.

The Yuthok Nyingthig contains a very extensive teaching on Karmamudra as a key point to achieve innate clear light experience. It is mentioned together with the Six Yogas in the chapter 'The Self-Arising Three Kayas of the Completion Stage'.

According to the Yuthok Nyingthig, the result of Karmamudra can lead to the attainment of the Rainbow Body.

Location	**Bliss and Emptiness**	
Throat Chakra	དགའ་བ། *(dga' ba)* Bliss	སྟོང་པ། *(stong pa)* Emptiness
Heart Chakra	མཆོག་དགའ། *(mchog dga')* Supreme Bliss	སྟོང་ཆེན། *(stong chen)* Great Emptiness
Navel Chakra	ཁྱད་པར་གྱི་དགའ་བ། *(khyad par gyi dga' ba)* Special Bliss	ཤིན་ཏུ་སྟོང་པ། *(shin tu stong pa)* Extreme Emptiness
Base Chakra	ལྷན་སྐྱེས་ཀྱི་དགའ་བ། *(ltan skyes kyi dga' ba)* Innate Bliss	རྣམ་པར་སྟོང་པ། *(rnam par stong pa)* Total Emptiness

Mahamudra

Mahamudra literally means 'Great Gesture', but is commonly translated as 'Great Seal'. It is one of the most advanced Tibetan meditation methods of the Vajrayana tradition, practiced by most of the Tibetan Tantric schools. It is a direct teaching about the true nature of mind. To achieve this ultimate state of mind and to cut off the root of samsara or constant suffering, Mahamudra clearly discloses the true nature of mind and all phenomena, their coexistence and also how to free oneself from dualism.

Mahamudra teaching is found both in the Sutra and Tantra traditions, without any conflicting views in terms of practice and is presented in different methods of meditation. Within sutra teachings such as the Prajnaparamita Sutras, it is conducted through Samatha and Vipassana meditation. The main presentation of Vajrayana Mahamudra is found in the Anuttarayoga Tantras where it is practiced by way of Tummo, Clear Light Yoga and Karmamudra.

In most Mahamudra teachings there are four important detailed practices which are called the ཕྱག་ཆེན་གྱི་རྣལ་འབྱོར་བཞི་ནི། *(phyag chen gyi rnal 'byor bzhi ni)* Four Yogas of Mahamudra. They can be understood as different states of mind that the practitioner gradually experiences. They basically equal the four points of Dzogchen's Trekchö, teaching on emptiness, hence Dzogchen and Mahamudra are considered parallel practices.

1. རྩེ་གཅིག་ *(rtse gcig)* Single Point

   In this stage the focused mind unified with understanding of emptiness brings bliss, clarity and a non-dualistic experience.

2. སྤྲོས་བྲལ་ *(spros bral)* Without Elaborations

   Upon continuing the single pointed meditation without attachment, this next stage is marked by the familiarization of the mind with its nature 'beyond mental constructs' which brings about the break down of dualistic thinking.

3. རོ་གཅིག་ *(ro gcig)* One Taste

   Further continuation of practice will lead the mind to experience all phenomena as essentially identical regarding the emptiness of their nature, thereby dissolving their appearance inseparably with the mind.

4. སྒོམ་མེད་ *(sgom med)* Without Meditation

   When this fourth state is reached, all types of mental activities become automatic meditation, as nothing further needs to be 'meditated upon'. Tilopa's six words of advice reflect this state:

- Don't recall (the past)
- Don't imagine (the future)
- Don't examine (the present)
- Don't analyze (try to reach conclusions)
- Don't control (try to make anything happen)
- Don't think (about dualism, just relax and rest)

As a continuation of Yuthok Nyingthig's foundational Tummo Yoga which aims at the transformation of the subtle body, རྩ *(rtsa 'khor)* channels and chakras, and subtle voice, རླུང *(rlung)* energy, the practice of Mahamudra deals with the mind, ཐིག་ལེ *(thig le)* essence drop, to complete the transformation into a Buddha's three kayas.

In contrast to Karmamudra, according to Yuthok, the teachings on Mahamudra are suitable for adult and elderly people. They are mentioned in the 19th chapter 'The Self-Arising Three Kayas' which is about Dzogrim, the completion stage.

Dzogchen

This practice, known as Mahasandhi or Atiyoga, is a direct meditation technique to reveal the ultimate nature of our mind. It is most commonly translated as 'The Great Perfection', a practice which greatly ends (samsara) as 'dzog' means end and 'chen' means great.

In the Yuthok Nyingthig the particular Dzogchen chapter is called རྫོགས་ཆེན་ངོ་སྤྲོད་འཁོར་འདས་རང་གྲོལ། *(rjogs chen ngo sprod lkhor 'das rang grol)* 'The Self-Liberation of Samsara-Nirvana'. It is a secret path for realizing the final rainbow body, the expression of the complete transformation and control over the elements of matter, energy and mind.

The two main Dzogchen practices are ཁྲེགས་ཆོད། *(khregs chod)* Break through Hardness and ཐོད་རྒལ། *(thod rgal)* Crossing the Skull.

As mentioned Trekchö consists of four points similar to the four yogas of Mahamudra, aiming at breaking through all logic and finding the true nature of emptiness in all phenomena, including the self and reality.

1. མེད་པ། *(med pa)* Non-Existence
   This point refers to the view that nothing exists independently or by itself, which makes all phenomena 'empty' of (independent) existence.

2. གཅིག་པུ། *(gcig pu)* Oneness
   Based on the aforementioned view Oneness expresses the realization that the self and reality are of the same empty nature, invalidating the differentiating view and dualistic grasping.
3. ཕྱལ་བ། *(phyal ba)* Omnipresence
   This nature of emptiness is beyond mind and matter.
4. ལྷུན་གྲུབ། *(lhun grub)* Spontaneous Manifestation
   Everything is spontaneously accomplished as it is.

Tögel shows how to realize the nature of the visionary and illusory manifestation of the self and all phenomena. It is a practice dealing with the subtle energies of lightness and darkness through which cosmic elemental powers are accumulated to develop the divine light body, also called rainbow body.

While the emphasis of Trekchö is on emptiness, the emphasis of Tögel is on appearance.

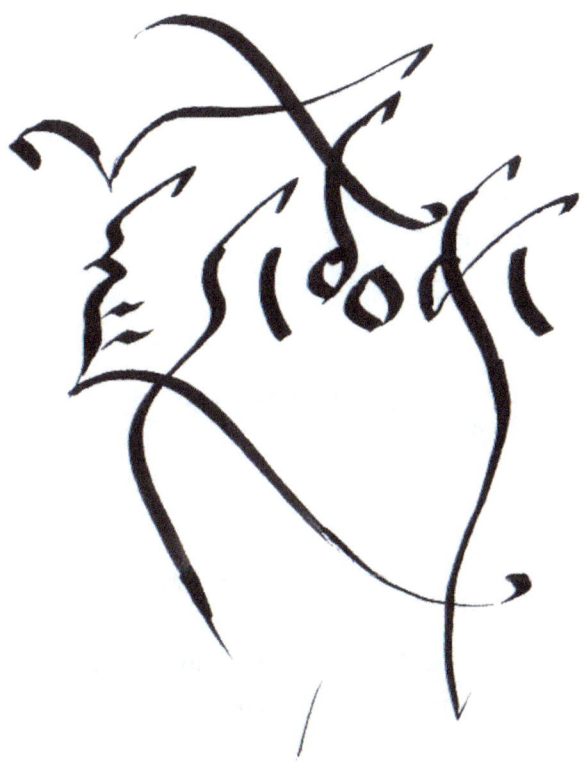

'Dzogchen', Tibetan calligraphy

Dzogchen

Additional Practices

Eliminating Obstacles	30
Signs of Practice	31
Action Practice	31
Long Life Practice	32
Fire Puja	32
Amulets	33
Pulse Practice	33
Protector Practice	33

The Yuthok Nyingthig contains various additional practices on the path to spiritual realization.

Eliminating Obstacles

Generally this practice of eliminating obstacles is meant to act against secret obstacle that hinder the study and practice of Yuthok Nyingthig and Tibetan medicine. It includes a daily visualization practice of Yuthok and the four dakinis.

Signs of Practice

Also called practice of eliminating inner obstacles, this chapter which describes the signs of practice is an important guide to progress on the spiritual path. Originally, it would be addressed only to the guru as a means of guiding the disciple instead of being given directly to the disciple.

Knowing the signs of a practice's positive result, the guru then gives the disciple instructions on how to eliminate obstacles when lacking or showing the wrong signs; or how to enhance the practice when showing correct signs. This subject therefore refers to inner obstacles.

Medical Action Practice

The action practice is also called practice of eliminating (the body's) outer obstacles. It is a comprised medical study with fifteen topics on causes, diagnosis and treatment of disorders of the three nyes pa[1], blood disorders, infectious diseases, metabolic diseases, pain, trauma, poisons etc. These are primarily meant for non-medical practitioners of Yuthok Nyingthig practices and are therefore

---

[1] Three principle energies which play a major role in the development of physical or mental disorders. They refer to རླུང་ *(rlung)* motion, མཁྲིས་པ་ *(mkhris pa)* burning energy, and བད་ཀན་ *(bad kan)* solid and liquid elements.

presented in a markedly simplified manner in comparison to the Four Tantras.

Long Life Practice

This practice shows one of the skillful means of the Vajrayana for prolonging the practitioner's lifespan in accordance with Guru Rinpoche's quote: "Of all activities, the first should be long life practice. If life is long, it can be virtuous. And the purpose of this life and the next can be achieved."

Yuthok Nyingthig's long life practice eliminates and prevents sickness in a simple and effective way.

Fire Puja

Fire pujas are one of the most powerful tantric rituals, performed for special reasons and to especially fulfill the Four Activities:

- Pacifying (famine, epidemics, natural disasters and war)
- Increasing (wisdom, longevity, merits and wealth)
- Controlling (one's emotions and the three realms)
- Destroying (insurmountable obstacles and negative forces)

The Yuthok Nyingthig contains a complete fire puja practice which is used for benefiting patients, families and communities.

Amulet
The text explains in detail how to create, activate and use this concise amulet to protect against and prevent negative energy influences.

Pulse Practice
These special instructions deal with the pulse reading practice and is therefore addressed to physicians of Traditional Tibetan Medicine in particular. In a spiritual retreat practitioners can enhance their pulse diagnosis abilities through the blessing of medicine goddesses and rishis.

Protector Practice
The medicine mahakalas or protectors are guardians of the Yuthok Nyingthig and the Four Tantras tradition. By doing the Protector practices, they then protect practitioners from worldly obstacles and spiritual misguidance, especially during difficult times.

The main medical protector, called Shanglon, is represented through two aspects: the Peaceful Shanglon with a retinue of five[1] who grants health and fortune, and the Wrathful Shanglon with a retinue of eight[2] who supports the spiritual practice.

---

[1] Nodjin Dondrubma, Zambhala, Namsei, Mahakala, Pancha Yakcha
[2] Mamo Ekazati, Zachen Rahula, Chechang Chumar, Shanpa Merutse, Damchen Dorje Legpa, Shanti Nagmo, Jigche Marmo, Habse Lekhan

གཞུ་ཐིག་སྙིང་ཐིག་གི་འགྲེལ་བའི་སྐོར།

COMMENTARIES

Zurkhar Nyamnyi Dorje

In the 15th century Zurkhar Nyamnyi Dorje, an accomplished spiritual master and physician of the lineage, edited the Yuthok Nyingthig together with The Four Medical Tantras upon having a vision of Yuthok asking him to clarify the texts and adding one guru yoga practice that Zurkhar had received as a terma. The reason being was that during that time some practitioners did not do the practice of the spiritual and medical teachings correctly.

Zurkhar also founded the Zur School, one of the two largest medical schools of Tibetan medicine. Its teachings, which combined spirituality and medicine, became the foundation of the Chagpori Medical College study and practice from the 17th century onwards and later of the Mentsee Khang in Lhasa.

Zurkhar Nyamnyi Dorje's clarifications include elaborations of shorter texts and instructions which up until then had only been transmitted orally. They became the foundation for the wood block prints of the Chagpori Medical College on which most of Yuthok Nyingthig editions are currently based. He also wrote a detailed commentary about the medical chapter of the Yuthok Nyingthig called *The Oral Teaching of One Billion Relics* with 416 chapters and various commentaries about the Four Tantras, many of them concerning the materia medica.

His Holiness the 5th Dalai Lama

Ngawang Lobsang Gyatso, the famous 5th Dalai Lama credited with the unification of Tibet in the 17th century, wrote several volumes on various fields not only on Buddhism but also medicine, astrology and other topics.

His minister, Desi Sangye Gyatso was a great supporter of Tibetan medicine and founded the Chapori Medical College in Lhasa, Tibet. He is the author of the famous *Blue Beryl*, a commentary containing approximately eighty thangkas (scroll paintings) on the most important reference work of Tibetan medicine, the *Four Tantras* by Yuthok.

Medical studies since the time of the 5th Dalai Lama to date are based on the Four Tantras. The main spiritual practice is Yuthok Nyingthig. Many monastic centers of Tibetan medicine, hospitals and clinics also do this spiritual practice.

The 5th Dalai Lama's commentaries related with the Yuthok Nyingthig include *The Wish-Fulfilling Tree*[1], a compiled ganapuja practiced and *The Wish-Fulfilling Tree of Dorje Dundul*[2], which is an additional protector practice introducing the peaceful Shanglon of Wealth.

---

[1] Yuthok Nyingthig Ganapuja, *The Wish-Fulfilling Tree of Sadhanas*, Sorig Press
[2] Part of *Yuthok Nyingthig Short Practice of Medical Protector Shanglon*, Sorig Press

Kongtrul Yönten Gyatso

The most famous commentary on the four guru yogas are the *'Notes on the Three-fold Outer, Inner, and Secret Practice of the Guru Sadhana'* by Kongtrul Yönten Gyatso. Born in 19th century in Eastern Tibet, he was trained from an early age in the classical sciences such as craftsmanship, logic, Sanskrit grammar, medicine and dharma. Subsequently, he later became an eminent Rime master recognized by all Buddhist schools due to his vast knowledge of the teachings regardless of their traditions as well as for his compilations of a hundred teaching volumes. Among these is the famous collection called *Rinchen Terzöd*[1], to which he added termas of Yuthok Nyingthig texts.

In his direct approach to the Yuthok Nyingthig practices, he joined the four guru yogas together into a four week retreat, in which the Outer Guru Yoga focuses on the guru as refuge field, the Inner Guru Yoga on the guru as Buddha, the Secret Guru Yoga on the guru as the Three Roots, and the Concise Guru Yoga on the guru as Vajrasattva Yab-yum. When it came to Yuthok Nyingthig's Dzogrim six yogas, Kongtrul Yönten Gyatso said that the explanation was "so clear, there was no need for any commentary".

---

[1] The Yuthok Nyingthig Guru Yogas and his commentary can be found in the *'Navel Chakra'* section, entitled the *'Deities of Knowable Amrita'*.

Karma Jigme Chökyi Senge

The 19th century Buddhist scholar Karma Jigme Chökyi Senge wrote several commentaries on different chapters which are now commonly used as foundation for Yuthok Nyingthig practices:
- *Mirror of Pristine Insight: A Pacifying Fire Offering*,
  the most commonly used text for Yuthok Nyingthig fire puja;
- *Puja of Blessing Medicine 'The Rishi's Mind Ornament'*,
  an additional puja meant for blessing medicine;
- *Joyful Ocean of Siddhis: An Instruction Manual for the Approach Practices of the Guru Sadhana*,
  a commentary on the Secret Guru Yoga;
- *Staircase for Traveling to the Pure Lands of the Three Kayas: A Detailed Explanation of the Aural Lineage*,
  a compiled practice of ganapuja;
- *The Clear Mirror of Nine Protectors*,
  a practice of the nine medical protectors.

He was one of the last and most important masters of Yuthok Nyingthig in the Chagpori College. He dedicated his life to teaching and giving transmissions in Central Tibet, thereby contributing greatly to the preservation of the teachings.

གཡུ་ཐོག་སྙིང་ཐིག་གི་ལོ་རྒྱུས།

HISTORY OF YUTHOK NYINGTHIG

Yuthok the Elder (729 - 854)

The greatest Tibetan physician was born on the fifteenth day of the Monkey month. According to legends, colorful rainbows appeared in the sky, and lights and music appeared spontaneously. His parents called him Yönten Gönpo, meaning 'Lord of Knowledge'.

At a young age, showing signs of extraordinary capacity and great compassion, he received visions of the Medicine Buddha and other enlightened beings. So, at the age of ten the King invited him to the Samye Palace where his medical expertise was tested against many other older Tibetan doctors. Yuthok unfalteringly showed an exceptional understanding of Traditional Tibetan Medicine, so much so that the King offered him the position of head doctor.

His journeys included several visits to India, Nepal, China and Odiyana, as well as some mysterious journeys to pure lands. Yuthok also studied at the Nalanda Monastery and received teachings in Astrology and Astronomy.

During his life he met accomplished spiritual masters and physicians, receiving teachings and transmissions of various traditions, such as the Dakini's practice from the ngakmo Tokpai Randrol, and various teachings, protection mantra and medicine from Guru Rinpoche. Through his dedicated spiritual practice he received further instructions, prophecies and teachings in many different visions.

At the age of forty-eight, Yuthok completed the '*Four Medical Tantras*' and wrote many other texts using them as educational or teaching texts for his disciples, thereby establishing the first standard medical educational system which still exists in Tibet to this day. Yuthok founded the first Tibetan medicine Centre for education called Menlung Gonpa Tanadug in Kongpo, where he taught every day. Amongst his thousand disciples, was the ngakmo Damey Mentsun, his most important female disciple.

He remained in meditation for three years and three months in a cave in the snow covered Lachi Mountain. When he returned to his hometown of Todlungkyina, the townsfolk joyfully offered him food, upon which he said 'I don't eat meat and I don't drink alcohol'. This was the first time he gave teachings on Ganapuja saying that without the base of a really stable meditation practice, nobody should eat meat or drink alcohol.

At the ripe old age of eighty-five, Yuthok married Dorje Tsomo with whom he had three sons to whom he later gave all his teachings.

After having written about thirty books on medicine, astrology and spiritual practices, he wrote his final medical book called Nyamtig Thongba Dontan and at the age of one hundred twenty gave his final teaching to his disciples. He told them that he would be soon going to the

Medicine Buddha's pure land where he would continue his activities.

On the fifteenth day of the Monkey month of the year of the Rat, the great Yuthok achieved the complete rainbow body with his wife Dorje Tsomo as well as their dog. Their bodies dissolved into light and rainbows. Natural sounds were heard, the earth moved, five colored lights were seen, a clear sky was experienced and it rained flowers for three whole months; all these are the signs of the highest realization.

Their three sons and their disciples built a liberation stupa and statues of Buddhas in memory of Yuthok.

Yuthok the Younger (1126 - 1202)

Born in the village of Goshi Rethang in Western Tibet, his father was Yuthok Khyungpo Dorje and his mother Pema Odenma. Yuthok came from a family lineage of royal court doctors whose origin can be traced to the time of King Lha Thothori (441 - 561).

At the age of eight he began to study a wide range of topics from medicine, Buddhism, and the arts and languages with his father and other teachers including Manjushri,. When he was fourteen he began traveling through Central Tibet where he met a Geshe called Roton Konchok Kyap who transmitted the *Four Tantras: the Essence of Ambrosia Secret Instruction* to Yuthok. Four years later he traveled to India for the first time where he studied the *Eight Branches of Healing, Somaradza* and other treaties on medicine with Paldan Trenwa. Upon his return to Tibet he set up a clinic and began teaching medicine. He then visited India a second time, where he received a teaching from the Dakini Mandarava which later became to be known as the *Yuthok Nyingthig, The Innermost Essence of Yuthok*.

It is said that he travelled to India six times. Not only did he become an unparalleled physician and was acclaimed as Yuthok Yönten Gönpo, meaning Yuthok 'Lord of All Qualities', but he also was an accomplished spiritual master, having had visions of Buddhas and shown exceptional signs.

One day, during his teachings at the Western Tibet governor's residence, fresh, golden Arura fruits fell within the walls of the residence for the duration of one hour. The people rushed to gather the fruits, fighting amongst themselves for it. Yuthok announced that if they had not angered the Goddess of Medicine with their greed, it would have rained other special medicines also. When his main disciple Sumtön Yeshe Zung asked Yuthok about the meaning of such special signs, Yuthok explained that the signs had three levels of meanings; an outer, an inner and a secret meaning. In an external or outer level, it indicated that there was no one in Tibet or India who could match Yuthok's knowledge. In an inner sense, it showed that Yuthok had attained the eight great powers (e.g. fast walking) and in a secret sense, it indicated that Yuthok was one and the same with the infinite mandalas of all Buddhas. In particular, these were signs that he was an emanation of the Buddha's doctor, of Padmasambhava, Ashvagosha, Padampa Sangye, Virupa, the famous doctor Kyebu Mela and in Tibet, of Srongtsen Gampo, Yuthok the elder and also of Gampopa.

Throughout all his life, Yuthok selflessly dedicated himself to others not only through teaching but also by donating the medicines he prepared to the sick and giving clothes to the needy.

Once, when Yuthok went to pay homage to a self-arisen statue of Buddha, a light emanated from the heart of the statue, resounding with the medicine Buddha mantra which spread everywhere. When the light dissolved, it entered Yuthok's head. He remained absorbed with his gaze lost in contemplation for a while and then called upon his student Sumtön Yeshe Zung Yuthok told him, 'You've been with me for twelve years. Now, if you have any doubts that have not been resolved please tell me now, I may soon depart for another land.' Sumtön was shocked and cried at the thought of his master passing away. 'You don't need to cry, I will live for sometime more. I told you this just to make you aware of the transitory nature of life'. Sumtön paid homage to the master and made a symbolic offering of the universe, then asked him for the ultimate teaching that would enable him to become a Buddha. In response,, Yuthok taught the Guru Yoga which is contained in the Yuthok Nyingthig.

It is said that at the age of seventy-six, Yuthok gathered his students for a final teaching before attaining the rainbow body and departing to Tanadug, the Medicine Buddha's pure land.

Yuthok's Song

When Yuthok the Younger reached the age of seventy-six, he summoned all his disciples to offer a teaching and presented them with many gifts. On that occasion, he briefly recounted his life story in the following song:

> Hey! Listen fortunate ones!
> Listen well, people of the world
> In particular, you who are gathered here
> Even though you have listened much before
> All those were meaningless illusory words
> Today you will listen to what is really meaningful
> Even though you have seen much before
> They were just designs of false & deceptive visions
> Today, that which you see will purify the two obscurations.
>
> If you do not know who I am
> I am the emissary of all Buddhas
> I am the refuge of all beings
> All the animate and inanimate world
> Is pervaded by my body, voice and mind.

The illusory form of this body
Is of the nature of a host of sacred deities
Its materiality is intrinsically pure
And like a rainbow it cannot be grasped, yet
Like the moon's reflection on the water, it appears everywhere.

The empty sound of my voice is the song of the echo
Reverberating with the sound of the eighty-four thousand Dharmas
It manifests as a rain of teaching for those who need to be guided
And sets all beings on the path that ripens and liberates.

In the clarity and emptiness of my mind, the ineffable authentic state
Bliss is omni pervasive, arising unceasingly and
Emptiness and compassion are undifferentiated
Hence, the phenomena created by mind are naturally liberated
Through the shortest instant of time.

In an instant I am a fully awakened Buddha
In an instant I travel to hundreds of Buddha fields
In an instant I encounter hundreds of Buddhas
In an instant I manifest hundreds of emanations
In an instant I guide hundreds of beings
And I accomplish the totalities and masteries.

With a faith that does not know uncertainties
Pray without having any doubt!
Even though the cataract of impure vision
Prevents you from seeing all these qualities of mine
In the ordinary perception shared by everyone.

I am the doctor who, with the medicine of skillful compassion
Cures the inner mental illness of the three emotions
The outer illness of the three humors, Wind, Bile and Phlegm
The title 'doctor' applies to me.

I explain the Buddhist canon and its commentaries by heart
With logic I overcome the challenges of fundamentalists
I issue the banner of victory of the Buddhist doctrine
The title 'scholar' applies to me.

I went to Sri Parvata and
Robbers created obstacles on my way
But with a gaze I paralyzed them all
The title 'siddha' applies to me.

On my way to Odiyana, flesh eating dakinis
Sent meteorites and lightning to strike me
I made the threatening gesture and all the dakinis collapsed
The title 'siddha' applies to me.

On my way to Ceylon
The boat fell apart in the midst of the waves
I flew like a bird and also saved my companions
The title 'siddha' applies to me.

When I went to the Kali forest
The vapor of venomous snakes spread like dark fog
I meditated on compassion and the fog quickly vanished
The title 'siddha' applies to me.

When I went to Persia
I encountered the army of the Mongols
So I penetrated the rocky mountains back and forth
The title 'siddha' applies to me.

When I visited Swayambhu
I competed with the Bönpos in magic
For half a day I remained sitting in space
The title 'siddha' applies to me.

I went from Bodhgaya to Tibet
Taking only a single day
Carrying a fresh flower as gift
The title 'siddha' applies to me.

At the place of Tshongdu Kormoru in Western Tibet
I prevented the sun from setting and
Caused a rain of Aruras, golden in color, to fall
The title 'siddha' applies to me.

It would be endless to recount all the events of my life
For one who has gained mind freedom
There are no disturbances caused by earth
Water, fire and wind, gods and demons etc
And by animate and inanimate enemies.

He flies in the sky swifter then birds
He dives in the waters with nothing to stop him
He penetrates mountains like a meteorite or lightning
In the midst of fire he is the fire god.

The beings of the degenerate age are of little merit
And few are those who meet and listen to me
Those who see, listen, think, touch me and have faith in me
Create the sprout of the spirit of enlightenment
Purify negativities accumulated throughout eons
Overcome obstacles and adverse condition of this life
Liberate themselves, liberate others, liberate both
And liberate all their followers.

I will connect to happiness even
Those who, harboring negative views, harm me
Hence, I will lead them from happiness to happiness
There is no doubt about this.

If you give up your heart and mind to me
Beseech me in a sincere way
Overcome your lack of faith and
Hope in me as a refuge throughout your life
Immediately your two obscurations will diminish
Upon meeting me in reality, in vision or in dream
I will reveal the path to the temporal and ultimate goal.

All of you present now and the students to come
My sons, and disciples remember this!
For the time being, my work of training beings in this world is complete
I will now go to the pure land of the Medicine Buddha.

Yuthok Nyingthig Lineage

1. སངས་རྒྱས་སྨན་བླ།
   (sangs rgyas sman bla) Medicine Buddha

2. གུ་རུ་པད་མ་འབྱུང་གནས།
   (gu ru pad ma 'byung gnas) Padmasambava (8th century)

3. གཡུ་ཐོག་ཡོན་ཏན་མགོན་པོ།
   (gyu thog yon tan mgon po) Yuthok Yönten Gönpo, the Elder (8th century)

4. མཁའ་འགྲོ་མ་དཔལ་ལྡན་ཕྲེང་བ།
   (mkha' 'gro ma dpal ldan phreng ba) Dakini Palden Tringwa

5. གཡུ་ཐོག་གསར་མ་ཡོན་ཏན་མགོན་པོ།
   (gyu thog gsar ma yon tan mgon po) Yuthok Yönten Gönpo, the Younger (12th century)

6. སུམ་སྟོན་ཡེ་ཤེས་གཟུངས།
   (sum ston ye shes gzungs) Sumtön Yeshe Zung (12th century)

7. གཞོན་ནུ་ཡེ་ཤེས།
   (gzhon nu ye shes) Zhönnu Yeshe (12th - 13th century)

8. ཞང་སྟོན་སངས་རྒྱས་ཡེ་ཤེས།
   (zhang ston sangs rgyas ye shes) Zhangtön Sangye Yeshe

9. མཁས་བཙུན་རིན་ཆེན་རྡོ་རྗེ།
   (mkhas btsun rin chen rdo rje) Khetsün Rinchen Dorje

10. བྲང་ཏི་དངོས་གྲུབ་རྒྱ་མཚོ།
    (brang ti dngos grub rgya mtsho) Drangti Ngödrup Gyatso

11. བྲང་ཏི་དཀོན་མཆོག་རྒྱལ་མཚན།
(brang ti dkon mchog rgyal mtchan) Drangti Könchok Gyeltsen

12. བྲང་ཏི་དཀོན་མཆོག་སྐྱབས།
(brang ti dkon mchog skyabs) Drangti Könchok Kyap *(14th century)*

13. ཟུལ་ཕུ་རིག་འཛིན་སྨན་མོ་རིན་ཆེན།
(zul phu rig 'dzin sman mo rin chen) Zülpu Rigzin Menmo Rinchen

14. རྣལ་འབྱོར་བསོད་ནམས་དབང་པོ།
(rnal 'byor bsod nams dbang po) Naljor Sonam Wangpo

15. རྣལ་འབྱོར་ཆེན་པོ།
(rnal 'byor chen po) Naljor Chenpo

16. རི་ཁྲོད་ཞིག་པོ།
(ri khrod zhig po) Ritrö Zhikpo

17. ཟུར་མཁར་མཉམ་ཉིད་རྡོ་རྗེ།
(zur mkhar mnyam nyid rdo rje) Zurkhar Nyamnyi Dorje *(15th century)*

18. དབྲག་དབོན་དཀོན་མཆོག་བཟང་པོ།
(dbrag dbon dkon mchog bzang po) Trakbön Könchok Zangpo

19. དཀོན་མཆོག་ནམ་མཁའ་རིན་ཆེན་དཔལ།
(dkon mchog nam mkha' rin chen dpal) Könchok Namkha Rinchen Pel

20. ལེགས་ལྡན་རྡོ་རྗེ།
(legs ldan rdo rje) Lekden Dorje

21. བཀྲ་ཤིས་སྟོབས་རྒྱལ།
(bkra shis stobs rgyal) Trashi Topgyel

22. བྱང་བདག་རིག་འཛིན་ངག་དབང་།
(byang bdag rig 'dzin ngag dbang) Jangdak Rigzin Ngakwang

23. ཟུར་ཆེན་ཆོས་དབྱིངས་རང་གྲོལ།
(zur chen chos dbyings rang grol) Zurchen Chöying Rangdröl

24. ངག་དབང་བློ་བཟང་རྒྱ་མཚོ།
(ngag dbang blo bzang rgya mtsho) Ngakwang Losang Gyatso

25. བློ་བཟང་ཚེ་དབང་།
(blo bzang tshe dbang) Losang Tsewang

26. ཀུན་བཟང་གྲོལ་མཆོག
(kun bzang grol mchog) Künzang Drölchok

27. ཆོས་འབྱོར་རྒྱལ་མཚོ།
(chos 'byor rgyal mtsho) Chöjor Gyeltso

28. རིག་འཛིན་བཟང་པོ།
(rig 'dzin bzang po) Rigzin Zangpo

29. པདྨ་གསང་བདག་བསྟན་འཛིན།
(pad ma gsang bngag bstan 'dzin) Padma Sangngak Tenzin

30. ཆོས་ཀྱི་རྒྱལ་མཚན།
(chos kyi rgyal mtshan) Chökyi Gyeltsen

31. མཐུ་སྟོབས་རྣམ་རྒྱལ།
(mthu stobs rnam rgyal) Tutop Namgyel

32. བསྟན་འཛིན་མཐུ་སྟོབས།
(bstan 'dzin mthu stobs) Tenzin Tutop

33. བྱམས་པ་བསྟན་འཕེལ།
(byams pa bstan 'phel) Jampa Tenpel

34. ཆོས་ཀྱི་སེང་གེ
(chos kyi seng ge) Chökyi Senge

35. རྟ་ཆུང་བླ་མ།
(rta chung bla ma) Tachung Lama

36. མཁན་ཆེན་ཁྲོ་རུ་ཚེ་རྣམ།
(mkhan chen khro ru tshe rnam) Khenchen Troru Tsenam[1]

37. མཁན་པོ་ཚུལ་ཁྲིམས་རྒྱལ་མཚན།
(mkhan po tshul khrims rgyal mtshan) Khenpo Tsültrim Gyeltsen[1]

38. མཁས་གྲུབ་མི་བསྐྱོད་ཚང་།
(mkhas grub mi bskyod tshang) Khedrup Michötsang (born 1929 in Amdo, Tibet)[2]

---

[1] Masters of Tibetan Medicine, Astrology and Buddhism from who Dr. Nida Chenagtsang received the full transmission and teaching in the 90s, while studying in the Lhasa Tibetan Medicine College (Editor's note)

[2] One of the most important living masters of the Yuthok Nyingthig of our time, from who Dr. Nida Chenagtsang received the transmission with the empowerment to teach and further transmit the Hayagriva Tantra and the Yuthok Nyingthig (Editor's note)

ཟུར་བཀོད།

APPENDICES

List of Yuthok Nyingthig Contents

Chapter	**Description**
1. The Iron Hook of Virtuous Qualities - The History	Historical introduction
2. The Supreme Empowerment of the Vast Expanse of Great Bliss	Long empowerment
3. The Condensed Essential Empowerment	Short empowerment
4. The Vajra-Knot of Samayas	Samayas
5. The Illuminating Lamp of the Direct Instructions on The Vajra-Knot of Samayas	Additional explanations on samayas
6. The Wish-Fulfilling Jewel of the Outer Practice	Outer Guru Yoga
7. The Source of Fulfilling all Wishes of the Inner Guru Yoga	Inner Guru Yoga
8. The Swift Guide for the Fortunate Individuals of the Secret Accomplishment	Secret Guru Yoga
9. The Wisdom-Wheel of the Concise Sadhana Practices of the Guru	Concise Guru Yoga
10. The Swift Speed Dakini	Dakini practice

Chapter	Description
11. The Speedy Dakini	Short dakini practice
12. The Condensed Realization of Visualizing the Five Families	Descriptions on the five family Buddhas
13. The Pond of Attainments, the Direct Instructions on the Inner Guru Yoga	Meditative study of the Four Tantras
14. The Path of Pleasurable Sensation, the Supreme Direct Instructions of the Secret Accomplishment	Simplified Secret Guru Yoga
15. The Secret Accomplishment Oral Transmission of the Sadhana of the Mahasiddha Mahaguna from the Blessing River of the Guru 'King of Medicine'.	Whispered tradition for the heart disciple
16. The Completely Satisfying Outer Torma Offering	Torma offering

Chapter	Description
17. The Completely Satisfying Outer Torma-Offering known as 'Source of All Accomplishments' from the Sadhana Blessing River of the Guru 'King of Medicine', the Activity Ritual Condensing the Meaning of Mother and Son, which is the Application of the Medicine Offering and Torma Offering for Swiftly Completing the Two Accumulations	Torma and medicine offering
18. The Net of Lights Fulfilling Offering of the Three Roots from the Blessing River	Fulfilling offering and confession
19. The Self-Arising Three Kayas of the Completion Stage	Dzogrim
20. The Root-Text of Yantras which is Clarifying the Darkness of Suffering	Yantra yoga base
21. The Direct Introduction to the Great Self Liberation of Samsara and Nirvana from the Cycle of Dharma Teachings The Blessing River	Dzogchen

Chapter	Description
22. Eliminating the Obstacles of Elemental Body Disorders	Medical study including 15 topics
23. Eliminating Obstacles of the Secret Obstructions of the Demonic Forces from the Blessing River	Practice of eliminating obstacles
24. The Jewel's Lamp which Clarifies the Signs of the Path	Explanations on the signs of practice
25. The Lineage Prayer for Guru Yoga	Praying to all gurus
26. The Blessing River	Meditation of guru yoga
27. Following the Experiences of One's Daily Practice from the Blessing River	Daily practice of guru yoga
28. The Ritual of Offering of Tormas	Torma offering
29. The One of Secret Form	Yuthok's Prayer
30. The Long Life Yoga Empowerment of Overcoming the Demon 'Lord of Death' from the Blessing River	Long life practice

Chapter	Description
31. The Long Life Empowerment of Overcoming the Demon 'Lord of Death'	Long life practice empowerment
32. The Complete and Swift Accomplishment through the Activities of the Fire Offerings	Fire puja
33. The Complete Protection from Fears through the Various Activities of Protection Wheels from the Blessing River	Protection amulet
34. The Bright Silver Mirror Divination of Pulse Reading	Pulse reading meditation
35. The Cycle of the Pulse Reading Son from the Blessing River	Short pulse reading empowerment
36. The Power and Strength of the Golden Mountain, the Skillful Means of Suppressing Negative Energy for Pulse Reading	Eliminating obstacles of pulse reading
37. Activities of the Silver Measure Sadhana of the Yellowish Rishi	Divination practice
38. The Wish-Fulfilling Jewel of Accomplishing the Rishi Divination	Long Outer Guru Yoga

Chapter	Description
39. The Illuminating Mirror of the Realization of Visualizing the Oath-Bound Protectors	Descriptions of the nine protectors
40. The Subjugation of the Wrathful Demons through the Fulfillment Offering to the Nine Oath-Bound Protectors	Protector practice
41. The Poisonous Force of the Threefold Razor of Granting Offering, Praise and Invocations to the Nine Protectors of the Teachings	Protector practice
42. The Drawing Forth of the Enemy's Red Life-Force through Wielding the Spinning Wrathful Wheel of the Sadhana of the Nine Oath-Bound Protectors from the Blessing River	Long protector practice
43. The Very Swift Blazing Flash of Lightning of Offering Petitions to the Dharma Protectors	Short protector practice
44. The Essence of the Life-Force, the Mantra Manual of the Nine Oath-Bound Protectors	Mantra list of the nine protectors

Explanations on Vajrayana

Origin of Tibetan Buddhism	66
Major Schools of Tibetan Buddhism	67
Chöd	68
Rime	69
Vajrayana System	69
Vajra Body	74
The Guru	76
Transmission System	77
Samayas	82
Base, Path and Result	84

Origin of Tibetan Buddhism

Buddhism was introduced to Tibet in the 7th century during the reign of the later named first 'Dharma King' Songtsen Gampo, founder of the Tibetan Empire, whose Chinese and Nepalese queens brought the first two Buddha statues to Tibet.

In the 8th century the Buddhist masters Padmasambhava and Shantarakshita were invited to establish Buddhism in Tibet by King Trisong Detsen who became known as the second Dharma King. According to the legends, Padmasambhava, called Guru Rinpoche in Tibet, subdued the spirits and negative forces of Tibet, therefore establishing Vajrayana Buddhism as the most suitable tradition. The translations of the Tripitaka and Outer Tantras during that time are considered the base of the later called Nyingma, ('old') tradition which would be the foundation of all following Tibetan Buddhist traditions.

The third Dharma King, King Relpacen, strongly supported Buddhism during his reign in the 9th century, after which suppression and eradication of Buddhism ensued.

A second wave of Buddhism once again flourished in the 11th century through the transmissions of Atisha, the Indian monk, who added the Mahayana and various Vajrayana teachings to the surviving yogic lineage of the Nyingma tradition.

Major Schools of Tibetan Buddhism

Atisha's arrival in the 11th century marked the second important transmission of 'new' schools called the Sarma tradition, complementing the 'old' Nyingma tradition. Tibetan Buddhism today has four main traditions:
- Nyingmapa, 'the Old Ones', founded in the 8th century by Guru Rinpoche and Shantarakshita. Their system is categorized by nine vehicles of which the highest is that known as Ati yoga or

Dzogchen. Termas are of particular significance to this tradition.

- Kagyupa, 'the Oral Lineage' which can be traced back to the Tibetan master Marpa in the 11th century, and includes famous practitioners such as Milarepa and Gampopa. This oral tradition is very much concerned with meditative experiences.
- Sakyapa, 'Grey Earth', representing a rather scholarly tradition. Headed by the Sakya Trizin 'Sakya Throne Holder', this tradition was founded by Khon Konchog Gyalpo in the 11th century. It promotes the Lamdre, containing the view that the result of its practice is contained within the path.
- Gelugpa, 'Way of Virtue', founded in the 14th century by the Buddhist scholar Je Tsongkhapa. This tradition is particularly known for its emphasis on logic and debate. Its spiritual head is the Ganden Tripa and its temporal one the HH Dalai Lama.

Chöd

The teachings of Chöd 'cutting [the ego]' or 'cutting the fear' combine the Prajnaparamita philosophy with specific meditation methods and tantric ritual. It was brought to Tibet by the Indian master Padampa Sangye at the end of the 11th century. The name Chöd is closely connected to Machig Labdron (1055 - 1149), founder of the Mahamudra Chöd Lineages, who accomplished the practice and substantially supported the development of these teachings. They were subsequently adopted by the four main schools.

Rime

The Rime movement was founded primarily through the masters Jamyang Khyentse Wangpo and Jamgon Kontrul Lodro Thaye in the 19th century in order to counteract suspicion and tension which was growing amongst the different Nyingma, Kagyu and Sakya traditions. As a result, it is responsible for the creation of a large number of scriptural compilations, such as the Rinchen Terdzöd. In addition the lineage heads and major figures of each tradition took teachings and empowerments from various schools and lineages.

Since the Yuthok Nyingthig is practiced in all traditions by the Buddhist ordinated and yogic practitioners it is considered part of Rime. Though its roots originate in the Nyingma tradition it encompasses features of both the old and the new schools.

Vajrayana System

Various different classifications are possible when describing Vajrayana :

1. Chronologically, Vajrayana can be considered as the third of the three 'turnings of the dharma wheel'; with Shakyamuni Buddha turning the first wheel when he gave his teachings of the Four Noble Truths[1], the base of today's Hinayana. The turning of the second wheel took place when he taught the Prajnaparamita Sutras at Vulture's Peak, leading to the Mahayana. Vajrayana's origination in the monastic Nalanda University is the third turning.
2. Teachings of Hinayana focus on becoming an ethical and moral being by protecting the mind from destructive emotions, while Mahayana emphasize Bodhicitta, the view dedicated to the liberation of all sentient beings. Vajrayana, the third wheel, introduces skillful means to achieve the latter goal.
3. In terms of methods Vajrayana or Tantrayana, the path of result, can be distinguished from the Sutrayana, path of accumulation. While the Sutrayana applies the method of renunciation, Vajrayana emphasizes transformation.

As Mahayana is based on the sutras of the Hinayana, the Vajrayana could likewise not exist without the twofold foundation of Hinayana and Mahayana.

---

[1] The Four Noble Truths are the nature of suffering, its cause, its cessation and the path to its cessation.

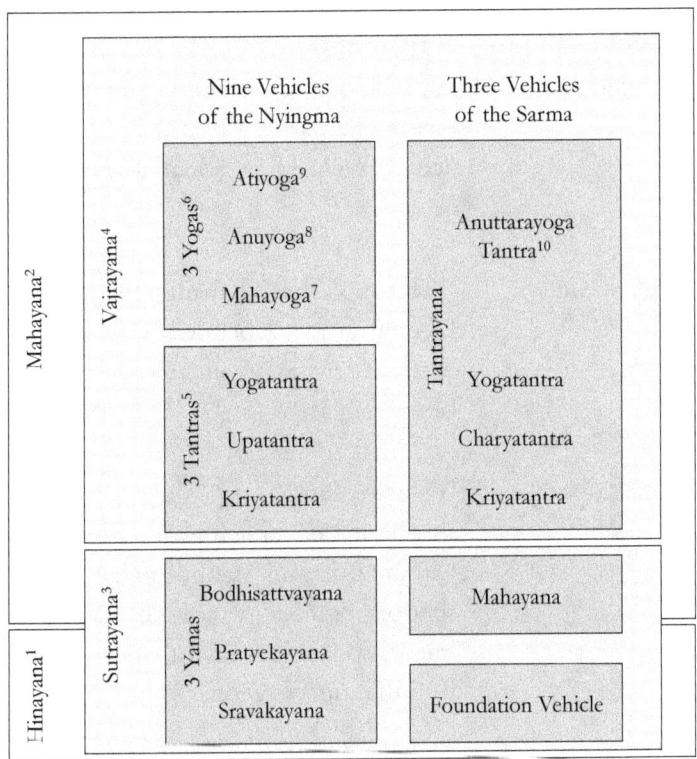

Overview of the Vajrayana system

[1] 'Smaller Vehicle' (Sanskr.)
[2] 'Great Vehicle' (Sanskr.)
[3] 'Vehicle of [Buddha's] Speech' (Sanskr.)
[4] 'Diamond Vehicle' (Sanskr.)
[5] Also called '3 Outer Tantras'
[6] Also called '3 Inner Tantras'
[7] Tib. Kyerim, antidote to anger
[8] Tib. Dzogrim, antidote to desire
[9] Tib. Dzogchen, result of the former yoga, antidote to ignorance
[10] Resulting in Mahamudra, Tib. Chagchen

Explanations on Vajrayana

Vehicle	Explanation
Sravakayana	'Vehicle of the Listeners', practice of virtues, Samatha, Vipassana; achievement of personal liberation as arhat
Pratyekayana	'Vehicle of the Self-Enlightened', meditation on dependent origination without relying on a teacher, becoming arhat
Bodhisattvayana	'Vehicle of the Bodhisattvas' (enlightened beings), Cittamantra and Madhyamaka schools, practice of compassion and meditation, achievement of Buddhahood in aeons
Kriyatantra	'Tantra of Activity', rituals of cleanliness, meditation on a deity, mantra recitation, attainment of Buddhahood in 7 lives
Upatantra/ Charyatantra	'Tantra of Practice', combining Kriya and Yogatantra

Vehicle	Explanation
Yogatantra	'Tantra of Realization', blessing of the guru, self visualization as deity, realization in 3 lives
Mahayoga	'The Great Yoga', visualization practice of Kyerim (generation stage), realization within one lifetime or during the bardo, antidote to anger
Anuyoga	'Subsequent Yoga', practice of Dzogrim (completion stage) focusing on the subtle anatomy, realization within one lifetime, antidote to desire
Atiyoga	'Ultimate Yoga', Trekchö ('cutting through'), view of rigpa, and Tögel ('direct leap'), working with clear light, instantaneous realization, antidote to ignorance
Anuttarayoga Tantra	'Highest Yoga Tantra', practice and result of Mahamudra (final of the Four Mudras*), considered equal to the Nyingma's Three Yogas

*The four mudras are found in the Anuttarayoga Tantra and Anuyoga, they are
1. དམ་ཚིག་ཕྱག་རྒྱ། *(dam tshig phyag rgya)* Samayamudra
2. ཆོས་ཀྱི་ཕྱག་རྒྱ། *(chos kyi phyag rgya)* Dharmamudra
3. ལས་ཀྱི་ཕྱག་རྒྱ། *(las kyi phyag rga)* Karmamudra
4. ཕྱག་རྒྱ་ཆེན་པོ། *(phyag rgya chen po)* Mahamudra

The foundation is Karmamudra, the union practice. Samayamudra, meditation on bliss, and Dharmamudra, keeping awareness, are supplemental. Mahamudra is the result, achievement of total wisdom.

Vajra Body

This refers to the 'Three Vajras' when working with channels and energies within Vajrayana Buddhism which does not only include our gross body, speech, mind ('Three Doors') but also a more subtle level of the triad. The realization of this subtle anatomy leads to the attainment of the Three Kayas, the realization of a perfectly enlightened being.

The subtle body consists of channels and chakras, in which the subtle speech moves as energy. The essence of this energy represents the subtle mind. These three are often metaphorically presented as house, person and jewels (རྩ། *(rtsa)* channels, རླུང་། *(rlung)* energy and ཐིག་ལེ། *(thig le)* essence drop).

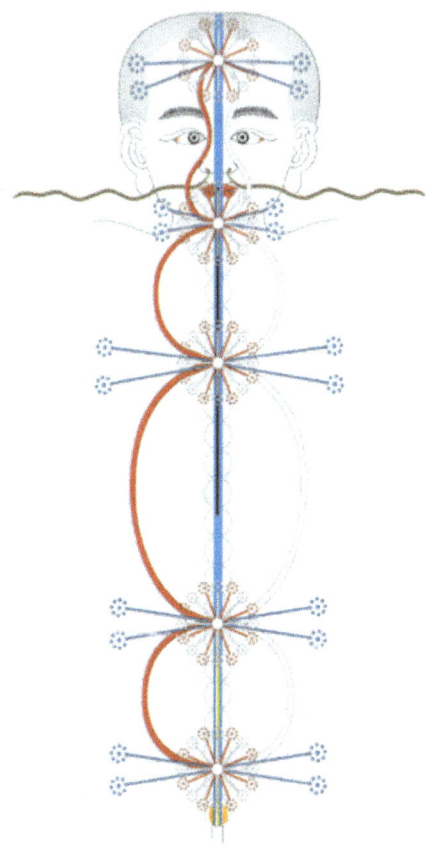

The Five Chakras from top are Head Chakra, Throat Chakra, Heart Chakra, Navel Chakra, Base Chakra.

Explanations on Vajrayana

The Guru

In Vajrayana traditions, the guru, in Tibetan called 'Lama', is regarded as Buddha, the root of one's own spiritual realization. Without the guru there will be no spiritual progress, no meditation experience and no wisdom. After what can be many years of careful evaluation and on mutual acceptance as guru and disciple respectively, the practitioner must have total devotion for the guru as well as absolute faith in the guru in order to receive his or her blessings.

In the Yuthok Nyingthig there are two main types of gurus, Appearance Symbol Gurus and True Self-Mind Gurus.

Appearance Symbol Gurus can be grouped into four categories:

- Root Guru, who reveals the true nature of your mind to you as that of Buddha;
- Lineage Guru, coming from the Vajradhara to your guru;
- Text Guru, also known as Never-Angry Black Guru, which is any text or book about the teachings of the Buddha and the enlightened ones;
- Self-Natured Guru, any phenomenon which can appear as subject to our five sense organs perfectly in the state of the union of appearance and emptiness, which ultimately is life itself.

The True Self-Mind Guru is the realization of our own nature whereby, at the foundational level, everything is created and projected by mind itself. Realizing this ultimate nature of mind, dualistic emotions will be self-liberated and the absolute realization takes place within mind itself, which the inner guru realizes is our own nature.

Transmission System

In Buddhism, teachings and practices are transmitted in various ways with different commitments and results, according to the divisions of the three vehicles, and even within one vehicle.

The complete Hinayana instructions as taught in the Tripitaka's Vinaya are usually received in a monastic context and come along with taking the pratimoksha vows, a set of several hundred codes. As ethical conduct, however, they are regarded as the basis of Buddhism with simplified sets of vows such as the Five or Eight Precepts also suggested to lay practitioners.

Mahayana teachings are usually transmitted freely both for monastic and lay practitioners. A voluntary set of Bodhisattva vows (several dozen), as found in the Avatamsaka Sutra, can be taken if practitioners wish to intensify their practice of Bodhicitta.

The transmission system in Vajrayana Buddhism is executed through a lineage of empowerments (sometimes also called 'initiations') which need to be received before the disciple is permitted to practice a particular tantra.

The guru performs the empowerment (usually of a practice cycle) as the disciple's own Buddha-nature reflected in the guru. The disciple must commit to specific samayas in order to preserve the spiritual link to the guru and ensure proper practice. To break a samaya is a serious downfall.

Various kinds of empowerments exist in the Vajrayana due to the different kinds of practices with different commitments and results of practice.

The Vajrayana transmission includes three steps before it is completed:

1. དབང་ *(dbang)* Wang[1]

    Wang is the ritual of the empowerment, literally translated as 'right' or 'power'. It gives the disciple permission to do a particular practice or cycle of practices.

2. ལུང་ *(lung)* Lung

    This is the reading or oral transmission, during which an authorized holder of the practice reads

---

[1] The Wang can be performed as complete རྩ་དབང་ *(rtsa dbang)* Root Empowerment in a long ritual or as དོན་དབང་ *(don dbang)* Essential Empowerment in a condensed form.

the original root text of the practice to the disciple who listens and has then created an auspicious connection with the practice.

3. བྱིད། *(khrid)* Trid

   The essential and most important part of a complete empowerment is the Trid, it consists of instructions and explanations on how to perform the practice. Without this the practice cannot be done properly.

Of these Wang and Trid are essential. Wang ripens the disciple's capacity of realization. Trid liberates them through instructing the actual application. Lung quotes the original teaching in order to ensure the instructions' authenticity.

Certain practices require their own particular empowerment due to their purpose or commitments, such as the ཚེ་དབང་། *(tshe dbang)* Long-Life-Empowerment[1], the སྲོག་གཏད། *(srog gtad)* Protector Empowerment[2], or the Yuthok Nyingthig specific དྲང་སྲོང་རིག་གཏད། *(drang srong rig gtad)* Rishi Empowerment[3].

---

[1] The Yuthok Nyingthig Long-Life-Practice is called 'Overcoming the Lord of Death'.
[2] The protector here refers to the medical mahakala Shanglon who vowed to protect the tradition of Yuthok Nyingthig and the Four Tantras.
[3] A unique empowerment found only in the Yuthok Nyingthig which requests the blessings of the rishis for enhancing medical abilities such as pulse reading

Explanations on Vajrayana

Empowerments of the Anuttarayoga Tantra

Empowerment	Vase	Secret	Wisdom	Word	All
Chakra Location	Head	Throat	Heart	Navel	Base
Syllable	OM	AH	HUNG	SHRI or SVA	SHRI or HA
Practice	Deity Yoga	Mantra Recitation	Karmamudra	Mahamudra	
Purification	Negative body karma	Negative speech karma	Negative mind karma	All negative karma	All negative karma
Blessing	Body	Speech	Mind	Knowledge or quality	Action or activity

Transformation	Ignorance	Desire	Anger	Pride	Jealousy
→	Dharma State Wisdom	Discriminating Wisdom	Mirror Like Wisdom	Wisdom of Equality	Accomplished Wisdom
Pure perception	Vision	Sound	Mind	Quality	Action
Realization	Nirmanakaya	Sambhogakaya	Dharmakaya	Kaya of Suchness	All kayas
Buddha	Vairocana	Amitabha	Medicine Buddha	Ratnasambhava	Hayagriva
Direction	East	West	Center	South	North

Explanations on Vajrayana

Empowerment of Anuttarayoga Tantras or the Three Inner Tantras (Three Yogas) authorize the disciple to be a certain deity, giving them the right to visualize him or herself as that deity - like a king being crowned and thus authorized to rule. The ritual process is divided into four parts, called the Four Empowerments:
- Vase Empowerment
- Secret Empowerment
- Wisdom Empowerment
- Word Empowerment

The Vase Empowerment symbolizes the purification of the disciple's body and channels, transforming it into a deity's body (achievement of Nirmanakaya). The Secret Empowerment purifies the disciple's speech and energy (achievement of Sambhogakaya). The Wisdom Empowerment purifies the mind and essence fluid (achievement of Dharmakaya). The Word Empowerment transforms the Three Doors and the Three Vajras and leads to the union of the three kayas, which is the realization of Suchness or the Clear Light state.

Samayas

The Samayas are a set of vows or commitment generating the bond between guru, disciple and tradition. They are formally created and obtained through the empowerment of a practice. Specific to Vajrayana Buddhism there are different levels and sets of Samayas. The Vajrayana samayas, including the Samayas of the Yuthok Nyingthig, for example, consist of fourteen root vows and twenty-five branch vows. Similarly, Traditional Tibetan Medicine originated from Buddha and comes with a set of oaths[1], hold onto by physicians as samayas are by spiritual practitioners.

They usually concern the actions of body, speech and mind and as such act as catalyzer for the spiritual progress. An intact Samaya will multiply benefits of a practice whereas a broken Samaya will not only destroy them all, but will lead to adverse and dire consequences. Through Samayas, positive and negative actions have a powerful karmic repercussion throughout many lifespans.

Some broken Samayas however may be repaired in time through means determined by the guru, such as fulfilling specific tasks, raising mindfulness, or doing the practice of purification and confession.

This is the reason why the guru and disciple should not choose each other carelessly, why transmissions

---

[1] The Medical Samayas are:
  1. Regard the guru as Buddha.
  2. Regard the guru's speech as Rishis' speech.
  3. Regard medical texts as Buddha's teachings.
  4. Regard colleagues and class mates as relatives.
  5. Regard patients as one's own children.
  6. Regard pus and blood like from the viewpoint of dogs and pigs.

should not be given and received without an adequate understanding, and why Vajrayana should not be practiced without commitment.

Base, Path and Result

The principle of development in spiritual realization according to Vajrayana is grounded on three points: base, path and result.

The base refers to the understanding of the vajra body. Studies concerning its channels and chakras, energies and essence are an integral part of every tantric practitioner's education.

The path refers to the practice of Kyerim and Dzogrim. While walking on the path three distinguished steps are to be taken:
1. ཐོས། *(thos)* listen
2. བསམ། *(bsam)* think
3. བསྒོམ། *(bsgom)* meditate

Through the process of listening (or reading) the disciple receives informative education, after which they have to go through the second step, which is an analytical process of thinking about the subject in order to reach a deep understanding of it. Doubts and confusion must be clari-

fied through discussion and questioning. Upon this favorable educational base and clear understanding, the third step which consists of meditation, will progress favorably. Hereby different signs will be indicative of the disciple's progress and they are to be known by the spiritual master; once again stressing the guru's indispensability in Vajrayana Buddhism. The progress can be:
- Gradual
- Unstable
- Instantaneous

Gradual realization is based on a stable foundation by practicing with patience in a constant and diligent manner. An unstable progress is marked by ups and downs of meditation experiences and signs. To attain realization it is particularly important not to be attached to the positive results that sometimes may appear. The instantaneous realization is only possible for very few practitioners with a perfect karma, created through determined and effortful practice in previous lives. The realization will still only happen through Guru Yoga.

The result refers to the achievement of the Three Kayas or the rainbow body.

In the unity of base, path and result, the Nyingma tradition especially emphasizes
- བལྟ། *(blta)* view,
- བསྒོམ། *(bsgom)* meditation,
- སྤྱོད། *(spyod)* behavior,
- འབྲས། *('bras)* fruit.

Herein the correct view of phenomena and spirituality forms the base. The path consists of meditation, which is the methodical practice of realizing this view, and action, the integration of this view into one's daily life behavior. The fruit will undoubtedly be achieved if the practitioner engages in correct meditation and behavior based on the correct view.

Glossary

Arura	Healing plant, also known as terminalia chebula or Chebulic Myrobalan, held by the Medicine Buddha in his right hand
Atisha	Indian Buddhist monk and scholar in the 10th and 11th century credited with introducing the second wave of Vajrayana Buddhism to Tibet
Avatamsaka Sutra	Sutra from the Sanskrit Canon, also called Flower Garland Sutra, explaining interdependent origination and the ten bhumis
Bardo	Transitional state after death and before the next life starts
Bhumi	Stages of progress on the path of a Bodhisattva to enlightenment, *see also Avatamsaka Sutra*

Bodhicitta	Literally awakened mind, compassionate mind striving for enlightenment for the benefit of all sentient beings
Bodhisattva	Enlightened being that dedicates all actions to benefit all sentient beings
Bumbachen	Literally vase breathing, tantric form of physical yoga
Chakra	Branching center of channels and energy in the body
Channel	Pathway of energy flow in the body
Circum-ambulation	Physical spiritual practice of walking around an object of veneration
Clear Light	Spiritual experience of the innate nature, also refers to the union of the Three Kayas
Completion Stage	*see Dzogrim*

Creation Stage	*see Kyerim*
Dakini	Female enlightened being, *see also Three Roots*
Dalai Lama	Highest master of Tibetan Buddhism
Deity	A Buddha as personal object of ones practice, *see also Three Roots*
Dependent origination	Central Buddhist concept that nothing exists by itself, complementary to emptiness, *see also Emptiness*
Deva	*see Deity*
Dharma	Sanskrit for phenomenon, Buddha dharma refers to the Buddhas teachings
Dharmakaya	Realization of subtle mind, *see also Three Kayas*
Dharmapala	Sanskrit for protector, *see also Protector*

Dorje Sempa	*see Vajrasattva*
Dzogrim	Also called Completion Stage, a perfecting phase of spiritual practice through yoga and meditation on the subtle anatomy
Emptiness	Central Buddhist concept that anything is devoid of independent existence, complementary to dependent origination, *see also Dependent origination*
Five Family Buddhas	Also called Five Dhyani Buddhas, Dharmakaya representations symbolizing the Five Wisdoms
Five Wisdoms	Series of five mental states attributed to the Dharmakaya, namely the Wisdom of Dharmadatu, the Mirror-like Wisdom, the Wisdom of Equanimity, the Differentiating Wisdom, the Accomplished Wisdom

Four Immeasurables	Series of virtuous mind states to be cultivated in Buddhism, namely loving-kindness, compassion, empathetic joy, equanimity
Four Noble Truths	Central Buddhist doctrine introduced as first teaching after Buddha Shakyamunis enlightenment, namely the nature of suffering, its cause, its cessation and the path to its cessation
Gampopa	A Tibetan physician and heart disciple of Milarepa
Ganapuja	Buddhist feast of offering and sometimes confession
Ganden Tripa	Official leader of the Gelug School of Tibetan Buddhism
Geshe	Tibetan Buddhist academic degree for monks and nuns

Guru Rinpoche	Also known as Second Buddha, introduced Vajrayana Buddhism to Tibet in the 8th century, founder of the Nyingma school
Hayagriva	Emanation of Avalokiteshvara or Medicine Buddha as wrathful deity
Heart disciple	Main disciple of a spiritual master or guru of a tradition
Intermediate state	*see Bardo*
Karma	Concept of body, speech and mind actions as the base for the samsaric cycle within the law of cause and effect
Karma Yoga	Practice of altruistic behavior in daily life
Kusali	Practice of mentally offering ones own body to four types of guests, simple form of Chöd

Kyerim	Also called Creation Stage, a development phase of spiritual practice, whose goal is to purify oneself being the deity
Lineage	*see Tantra*
Loka	Samsaric realms, namely of gods, asuras, humans, animals, pretas, hell beings
Mahakala	One of the main Dharmapalas in Vajrayana Buddhism
Mandala	Usually round or square Buddhist symbol, representing the universe
Manjushri	Enlightened being associated with wisdom
Mantra	Literally 'mind protection', a syllable or group of syllables with hidden (spiritual) power contained in its vibration

Medicine Buddha	Buddha of healing and medicine, introduced in the Medicine Buddha Sutra by Shakyamuni Buddha
Milarepa	Tibets most famous yogi, heart disciple of Marpa, foremost student of Naropa
Mudra	Literally means gesture, usually performed with hands by Buddhas to express a particular symbolic meaning
Nalanda University	One of the worlds first international residential and most famous Buddhist universities existing from the 5th to almost the 13th century in India with more than 10,000 students and teachers in an area comprised of 150,000 square meters, owning up to 200 villages at times
Naropa	Heart disciple of Tilopa, credited with the creation of the Six Yogas, *see also Tilopa*

Ngakpa, ngakmo	*see Yogi, yogini*
Niguma	Female equivalent of Naropa, sometimes credited as his sister, credited with the creation of the Six Yogas, *see also Naropa*
Nirmanakaya	Realization of subtle body, *see also Three Kayas*
Nirvana	Liberation of the mind from suffering
Odiyana	Guru Rinpoches place of origin
Padmasambhava	*see Guru Rinpoche*
Prajnaparamita Sutras	Collection of sutras from the Sanskrit Canon dealing with the concept of Prajnaparamita, the Perfection of Wisdom, as an important part of a Bodhisattvas path, stating that phenomena exist only in the mind

Prostration	Physical spiritual practice of bowing or lying down before an object of veneration
Protector	Emanation of Buddha appearing as wrathful deity to defend and guard the dharma
Puja	*see Ganapuja*
Rainbow body	Expression of complete realization, result of the Dzogchen practice of Tögel
Refuge field	Also called refuge tree, visualized or painted representation of a Buddhist traditions lineage gurus and transmissions
Retreat	A certain time of solitude or community experience dedicated solely to spiritual practice
Rishi, rishika	A male, female sage who has attained realization

Sadhana	Spiritual practice with the goal of reaching enlightenment
Samatha	Calm abiding meditation for pacifying the mind and increasing its concentration, foundation for Insight meditation
Sambhogakaya	Realization of subtle speech or energy, *see also Three Kayas*
Samsara	Repeating cycle of birth, life, death and rebirth within the six lokas
Sangha	Monastic community of ordained Buddhist monks or nuns, *see also Three Jewels*
Shakyamuni Buddha	Historical Buddha and founder of Buddhism

Shantarakshita	Famous abbot and scholar of the Nalanda University in 8th century India, who together with Guru Rinpoche introduced Vajrayana Buddhism to Tibet
Somaradza	Famous Tibetan Medicine text by the translator Vairotsana, 8th century
Sowa Rigpa	Literally means Healing Science, vernacular name of Traditional Tibetan Medicine
Stupa	A building or structure containing Buddhist relics, symbolizing the Buddhas body
Sumtön Yeshe Zung	Yuthok's heart disciple
Sutra	Buddha's speech or teaching, *see also Tripitaka*
Tanadug	Pure land or garden of the Medicine Buddha

Tantra	Literally means lineage of teaching, system of transmission of a tradition's teachings; if from an unbroken lineage, it preserves the purity and originality of the teaching
Terma	Literally means hidden treasure, refers to secret spiritual teachings hidden away by Guru Rinpoche or his consort Yeshe Tsogyal in the 8th century to be discovered in the future by so called tertöns
Thangka	Painting usually depicting a Buddhist deity, scene, or mandala
Three Doors	Body, speech and mind
Three Jewels	Object of refuge for Buddhists, consisting of Buddha, Dharma, Sangha

Three Kayas	Nirmanakaya, Sambhogakaya, Dharmakaya, realizations of the vajra body of a completely enlightened being
Three mental poisons	Attachment, hatred, ignorance
Three Roots	Object of refuge for tantric Buddhist practitioners, consisting of Guru, Deva, Dakini
Three Vajras	Vajra body, vajra speech, vajra mind
Tilopa	A tantric practitioner and mahasiddha who developed the mahamudra method, his famous Six Words of Advice was a teaching to his heart disciple Naropa
Torma	A figure made of flour and butter used in tantric rituals or as offerings in Vajrayana Buddhism

Tripitaka	Three categories (literally baskets) of texts, namely Sutras, Abhidharma, Vinaya, constituting the foundational Buddhist canon, also called Pali Canon
Tsongkhapa	Famous teacher of Tibetan Buddhism, credited with the formation of the Gelug school
Vajrasattva	Enlightened being closely associated with the practice of purification
Vajravarahi	Wrathful female deity, consort of Chakrasamvara or Hayagriva, important figure in the Kagyu school
Vinaya	*see Tripitaka*
Vipassana	Insight meditation leading to spiritual realization, based on Samatha
Yabyum	Tibetan for union or in union
Yantra Yoga	Yoga of Movement, *see also Yoga*

Yidam	*see Deity*
Yoga	Literally Achievement of Truth, spiritual practice of body, speech or mind
Yogi, yogini	Male, female practitioner of yoga, *see also Yoga*

Bibliography

Tibetan Sources

གཡུ་ཐོག་སྙིང་ཐིག་བླ་སྒྲུབ་ཕྱག་བཞལ་མུན་སེལ། ཕྱགས་པོ་རི། ཕྱགས་པོ་རིའི་དཔར་ཁང་། ཤིང་དཔར་མ།

གཡུ་ཐོག་སྙིང་ཐིག ཕྱགས་མང་ཞིབ་འཇུག་ཁང་། པེ་ཅིང་མི་རིགས་དཔེ་སྐྲུན་ཁང་། ཕྱགས་དཔར་མ།

གཡུ་ཐོག་སྙིང་ཐིག་ཚོག ང་རམས་མ་ལ་སྨན་རྩིས་ཁང་། ང་རམས་མ་ལ་སྨན་རྩིས་ཁང་། ཕྱགས་དཔར་མ།

གཡུ་ཐོག་སྙིང་ཐིག ཨ་དུ་ར་སྨན་གྱི་ཚོགས་པ། མི་རིགས་དཔེ་སྐྲུན་ཁང་། ཕྱགས་དཔར་མ།

English Sources

Chenagtsang N. *The Tibetan Art of Good Karma: The Hidden Treasure of the Turquoise Way.* Sorig Publications Australia, 2011

Parfionovitch Y, Dorje G. *Tibetan Medical Paintings: Illustrations to the Blue Beryl, Treatise of Sangye Gyamtso (1653 - 1705: Plates and Text).* New York, Harry N Abrams, 1992.

Yeshe Tsogyal. *The Lotus-Born: The Life Story of Padmasambhava*. Hong Kong, Rangjung Yeshe Publications, 2004.

Namkhai Nyingpo, Gyalwa Changchub. *Lady of the Lotus-Born: The Life and Enlightenment of Yeshe Tsogyal*, Boston, Shambala Publications, 1999.

The Life of Shabkar: The Autobiography of a Tibetan Yogin. Translated by Matthieu Ricard. Ithaca, Snow Lions Publications, 2001.

Index

A

Amulet	2, 6, 33
Anuyoga, see Nine Vehicles	13, 16, 73, 74
Appearance Symbol Guru, see Guru	76
Lineage Guru	76
Root Guru	76
Self-Natured Guru	76
Text Guru	76
Arura	46, 87
Astrology	42, 58
Astronomy	42
Atisha	67, 87
Atiyoga, see Nine Vehicles	27, 73
Avatamsaka Sutra	77, 87
Aversion, see Hatred	20
Awareness	7

B

Bardo	1, 5, 16, 18, 19, 20, 73, 87, 92
Bardo Yoga	1, 5, 16, 20
Bhumi	87
Bliss, see Four Blisses	23, 49, 60
Blue Beryl	37, 103
Bodhicitta	8, 9, 70, 77, 88
Bodhisattva	7, 77, 87, 88
Bodhisattvayana, see Nine Vehicles	72
Break through Hardness, see Dzogchen	27
Buddha	7, 9, 10, 11, 12, 14, 26, 38, 46, 47, 50, 66, 76, 83, 89, 91, 92, 94, 96, 98, 99
Historical Buddha	7, 97
Buddhahood, see Nirvana	17, 72
Buddhism	12, 37, 45, 58, 66, 67, 74, 77, 78, 83, 85, 87, 91, 92, 93, 97, 98, 100
Mahayana	67, 70, 77
Tibetan Buddhism	2, 66, 67, 89, 91, 101
Vajrayana	2, 3, 12, 24, 32, 66, 67, 69, 70, 74, 76, 78, 83, 84, 85, 87, 92, 93, 98, 100
Bumbachen	19, 88

C

Chagpori	36, 39
Chakra, see Five Chakras	23, 38, 88
Channel	88
Charyatantra, see Three Vehicles	72
Chöd	2, 66, 68, 92
Circumambulation	9
Cittamantra	72
Clear Light	1, 5, 14, 16, 18, 19, 24, 82, 88
Clear Light Yoga	1, 5, 16, 18, 19, 24
Common Ngöndro, see Ngöndro	1, 5, 7, 8
Compassion	11, 42, 49, 50, 52, 72, 91
Concise Guru Yoga, see Guru Yoga	1, 5, 12, 14, 38, 60
Consciousness	21
Controlling, see Four Activities	32

Creation stage, see Kyerim   5, 89, 93
Crossing the Skull, see Dzogchen   27

D

Dakini Practice   1, 5, 12, 13, 15, 42, 45, 55, 60, 61, 89, 100
Dakini, see Three Roots   1, 5, 12, 15
Dalai Lama   2, 37, 68, 89
    Ngawang Lobsang Gyatso   37
Death   63, 64, 79
Deity, see Three Roots   12, 89, 102
Dependent origination   89, 90
Desi Sangye Gyatso   37
Destroying, see Four Activities   32
Deva, see Three Roots   12, 13, 89, 100
Dharma   6, 8, 9, 12, 62, 65, 66, 67, 89, 99
Dharma King   66, 67
    Replacen   67
    Songtsen Gampo   66
    Trisong Detsen   66
Dharmakaya   82, 89, 90, 100
Dharmamudra, see Four Mudras   74
Dharmapala   89
Donations   10
Dorje Sempa, see Vajrasattva   9, 90
Dream Yoga   1, 5, 16, 18, 19
Dzogchen   1, 5, 25, 27, 62, 68, 73, 96
    Break through Hardness   27
    Crossing the Skull   27
    Tögel   28, 73, 96
    Trekchö   25, 27, 28, 73
Dzogrim   1, 5, 13, 14, 16, 17, 18, 22, 26, 38, 62, 73, 84, 88, 90

E

Eliminating Obstacles, see Practice   2, 5, 30, 63
Emanation, see Buddha   92, 96
Empowerment   60, 63, 64, 78, 82
    Long-Life-Empowerment   79
    Protector Empowerment   79
    Rishi Empowerment   79
    Trid   79
    Wang   78, 79
Emptiness, see Impermanence   23, 49, 89, 90
Energy, see Rlung   64
Enlightenment, see Nirvana   104

F

Fire Puja   2, 6, 30, 32
Five Family Buddhas   90
Five Wisdoms   90
Four Activities   13, 32
    Controlling   32
    Destroying   32
    Increasing   32
    Pacifying   32, 39
Four Blisses   22
    Bliss   23, 49, 60
    Innate Bliss   23
    Special Bliss   23
    Supreme Bliss   23
Four Empowerments   13, 82
Four Immeasurables   9, 91
Four Mudras   73
Four Noble Truths   70, 91

Four Tantras, see Gyud shi 7, 14, 32, 33, 36, 37, 45, 61, 79
Four Yogas, see Mahamudra 24

G

Gampopa 46, 68, 91
Ganapuja 37, 43, 91, 96
Ganden Tripa 68, 91
Gelug, see Sarma 91, 101
Geshe 45, 91
Great Perfection, see Dzogchen 5, 27
Guru 3, 6, 12, 13, 32, 38, 39, 42, 47, 60, 61, 62, 63, 66, 67, 76, 85, 92, 95, 98, 99, 100, 2
Guru Rinpoche 32, 42, 67, 92, 95, 98, 99
Guru Yoga 12, 13, 14, 15, 32, 36, 38, 42, 47, 63, 67, 85, 92, 95, 98, 99
   Concise Guru Yoga 1, 5, 12, 14, 38, 60
   Inner Guru Yoga 1, 5, 12, 14, 38, 60, 61
   Outer Guru Yoga 1, 5, 12, 13, 38, 60, 64
   Secret Guru Yoga 1, 5, 12, 14, 38, 39, 60, 61
Guru, see Three Roots 12, 13, 38, 47, 63, 85

H

Hayagriva 14, 58, 92, 101
Heart disciple 92, 94
Hinayana 70, 77
Historical Buddha, see Buddha 97

I

Ignorance 19
Illusory Body Yoga 1, 5, 16, 18, 20
Impermanence 8
Increasing, see Four Activities 32
Innate Bliss, see Four Blisses 23
Inner Guru Yoga, see Guru Yoga 1, 5, 12, 14, 38, 60, 61
Inner Tantra, see Tantra 13, 82
Intermediate state 92

J

Jamyang Khyentse Wangpo 69

K

Kagyu, see Sarma 16, 69, 101
Karma 2, 9, 10, 18, 22, 39, 85, 92, 103
Karma Jigme Chökyi Senge 2, 39
Karmamudra 1, 5, 18, 22, 23, 24, 26, 74
Karmamudra, see Four Mudras 1, 5, 18, 22, 23, 24, 26, 74
Kindness 9, 11
Kongtrul Yönten Gyatso 2, 38
Kriyatantra, see Nine Vehicles 72
Kusali practice, see Practice 9
Kyerim 1, 5, 12, 14, 73, 84, 89, 93

L

Lama, see Guru 58, 76
Law of cause and effect 9, 92

Lhasa	36, 37, 58
Liberation, see Nirvana	21, 62, 95
Lineage	2, 39, 55, 63, 68, 76, 93
Lineage Guru, see Appearance Symbol Guru	76
Loka	93
Long Life Practice, see Practice	2, 6, 30, 32
Long-Life-Empowerment, see Empowerment	79

M

Machig Labdron	68
Madhyamaka	72
Mahakala	34, 93
Mahamudra	1, 5, 24, 26, 27, 73, 74
Mahamudra, see Four Mudras	1, 5, 24, 26, 27, 69, 73, 74
Mahasandhi, see Dzogchen	1, 5, 24, 26, 27, 69, 73, 74
Mahayana, see Buddhism	27
Mahayana, see Three Vehicles	67, 70, 77
Mahayoga, see Nine Vehicles	67, 70, 77
Mandala	8, 9, 13, 93, 99
Mandala offering	8, 9
Mandala offering, see Mandala	8, 9
Manjushri	45, 93
Mantra, see Tantra	65, 93, 115
Medical Action Practice, see Practice	2, 6, 31
Medicine Buddha	14, 21, 42, 44, 47, 54, 55, 87, 92, 94, 98
Meditation, see Practice	63
Mentsee Khang	36
Milarepa	68, 91, 94
Mind	39
Mudra	94

N

Nalanda University	70, 94, 98
Naropa	16, 94, 95, 100
Never-Angry Black Guru, see Appearance Symbol Guru	76
Ngakpa, see Tantra	95, 115
Ngawang Lobsang Gyatso, see Dalai Lama	37
Ngöndro	1, 5, 7, 8
Common Ngöndro	1, 5, 7, 8
Routin Ngöndro	1, 5, 7, 8, 10
Uncommon Ngöndro	1, 5, 7, 8, 9, 10
Niguma	16, 95
Nine Vehicles	2
Nirmanakaya	82, 95, 100
Nirvana	9, 62, 95
Non-Existence, see Trekchö	27
Nyingma	16, 67, 69, 73, 86, 92, 2

O

Odiyana	42, 51, 95
Offering	6, 39, 47, 61, 62, 63, 65, 91, 92
Omnipresence, see Trekchö	28
One Taste, see Mahamudra	25
Oneness, see Trekchö	28
Outer Guru Yoga, see Guru Yoga	1, 5, 12, 13, 38, 60, 64
Outer Tantra, see Tantra	12, 67

P

Pacifying, see Four Activities   32, 39
Padampa Sangye   46, 68
Padmasambhava, see Guru Rinpoche 46, 66, 95, 104
Path   3, 5, 8, 61, 63, 66, 84
Phowa   1, 5, 16, 18, 21
Practice   2, 5, 6, 7, 5, 6, 7, 9, 10, 12, 13, 14, 15, 16, 17, 18, 19, 21, 22, 24, 25, 26, 27, 28, 30, 31, 32, 33, 36, 37, 38, 39, 42, 43, 60, 63, 64, 65, 68, 69, 72, 73, 74, 77, 78, 79, 83, 84, 85, 86, 89, 92, 96, 101, 2
   Eliminating Obstacles 2, 5, 30, 63
   Karma yoga   10, 92
   Kusali practice   9
   Long Life Practice   2, 6, 30, 32
   Preliminary practice   1, 5, 7, 8
   Protector Practice   2, 6, 30, 33
   Pulse practice   2, 6, 30, 33
   Spiritual practice 5, 6, 7, 8, 19, 20, 21, 24, 32, 34, 37, 42, 43, 76, 83, 84, 86, 88, 90, 93, 96, 97, 100, 102, 2
Prajnaparamita Sutra   24, 70, 95
Pratyekayana, see Nine Vehicles   72
Prostration   8, 9, 96
Protector Empowerment, see Empowerment   9, 96
Protector Practice, see Practice   2, 6, 30, 33, 37, 65, 79, 89, 96
Protector, see Mahakala   79
Puja, see Ganapuja   2, 6, 30, 33
Pulse practice, see Practice   2, 6, 30, 32, 39, 96
Purification   39

R

Rainbow body   96
Refuge 8, 9, 12, 13, 38, 48, 54, 96, 99, 100
Refuge field, see Three Roots   96
Relpacen, see Dharma King   67
Retreat, see Practice   96
Rime   3, 38, 66, 69
Rinchen Terzöd   38
Rishi   39, 64, 79, 96
Rishi Empowerment, see Empowerment 79
Root Guru, see Appearance Symbol Guru 76
Routine Ngöndro, see Ngöndro 1, 5, 7, 8, 10

S

Sadhana 6, 37, 38, 39, 60, 61, 62, 64, 65, 97, 2
Sakya, see Sarma   68, 69
Samatha, see Practice 12, 24, 72, 97, 101
Samaya   83
Samayamudra, see Four Mudras   74
Sambhogakaya, see Three Kayas 20, 82, 97, 100
Samsara   9, 19, 24, 27, 62, 97
Samye   42
Sangha   9, 12, 97, 99

Index

Sanskrit	38, 87, 89, 95
Sarma	67, 2
Seal, see Mudra	5, 24
Secret Empowerment, see Four Empowerments	82
Secret Guru Yoga, see Guru Yoga	1, 5, 12, 14, 38, 39, 60, 61
Self-Mind Guru, see Guru	76, 77
Self-Natured Guru, see Appearance Symbol Guru	76
Sentient being	11, 70, 88
Shakyamuni Buddha	70, 94, 97
Shanglon	33, 37, 79
Shantarakshita	66, 67, 98
Signs of Practice, see Practice	2, 5, 30, 31
Single Point, see Mahamudra	25
Six Yogas	16, 17, 18, 19, 22, 94, 95
Somaradza	45, 98
Songtsen Gampo, see Dharma King	66
Sowa Rigpa, see Tibetan medicine	7, 98
Special Bliss, see Four Blisses	23
Spiritual practice, see Practice	97
Spontaneous Manifestation, see Trekchö	28
Sravakayana, see Nine Vehicles	72
Stupa	98
Suchness	82
Sumtön Yeshe Zung	46, 47, 55, 98
Supreme Bliss, see Four Blisses	23
Sutra	24, 87, 94, 98

T

Tanadug, see Pure Land	43, 47, 98
Tantra	17, 24, 58, 72, 73, 74, 78, 93, 99
Tantrayana, see Three Vehicles	70
Terma	99
Text Guru, see Appearance Symbol Guru	76
Thangka	99
Three Doors	74, 82, 99
Three Jewels	9, 12, 97, 99
Three Kayas	18, 22, 26, 39, 62, 74, 85, 88, 89, 95, 97, 100
Three mental poisons	100
Three Roots	12, 14, 15, 38, 62, 89, 100
Dakini	1, 5, 12, 13, 15, 42, 45, 55, 60, 61, 89, 100
Deva	12, 13, 89, 100, 102
Guru	3, 6, 12, 13, 14, 15, 31, 32, 36, 38, 39, 42, 47, 60, 61, 62, 63, 66, 67, 73, 76, 77, 78, 82, 83, 85, 92, 95, 98, 99, 100, 2
Three Vajras	17, 74, 82, 100
Three Vehicles	2
Tibetan Buddhism, see Buddhism	2, 66, 67, 89, 91, 101
Tibetan medicine	5, 7, 8, 30, 33, 36, 37, 42, 43, 83, 98, 115, 2
Tilopa	25, 94, 100
Tögel, see Dzogchen	28, 73, 96
Torma	61, 62, 63, 100
Traditional Tibetan Medicine, see Tibetan medicine	5, 7, 33, 42, 83, 98, 115, 2
Transmission, see Empowerment	3, 61, 66, 77
Trekchö, see Dzogchen	25, 27, 28, 73
Trid, see Empowerment	79

Tripitaka 67, 77, 98, 101
Trisong Detsen, see Dharma King 66
Tsongkhapa 68, 101
Tummo 1, 5, 16, 18, 19, 20, 22, 24, 26

U

Uncommon Ngöndro, see Ngöndro 1, 5, 7, 8, 9, 10
Union 20
Upatantra, see Nine Vehicles 72

V

Vajrasattva 9, 14, 38, 90, 101
Vajravarahi 14, 101
Vajrayana, see Buddhism 2, 3, 12, 24, 32, 66, 67, 69, 70, 74, 76, 78, 83, 84, 85, 87, 92, 93, 98, 100
Vase Empowerment, see Four Empowerments 82
Vinaya, see Tripitaka 77, 101
Vipassana, see Practice 24, 72, 101
Virupa 46

W

Wang, see Empowerment 78, 79
Wisdom 82, 90, 95
Wisdom Empowerment, see Four Empowerments 82
Without Elaborations, see Mahamudra 25
Without Meditation, see Mahamudra 21, 25

Word Empowerment, see Four Empowerments 82

Y

Yabyum, see Union 101
Yantra Yoga 101
Yidam, see Three Roots 12, 102
Yoga 1, 5, 10, 12, 13, 16, 18, 19, 20, 24, 26, 63, 73, 92, 101, 102, 115
Yogatantra, see Nine Vehicles 72, 73
Yogi 95, 102
Yuthok Nyingthig 2, 5, 7, 8, 5, 7, 8, 9, 10, 12, 13, 15, 18, 22, 23, 26, 27, 30, 31, 32, 33, 36, 37, 38, 39, 45, 47, 55, 58, 60, 69, 76, 79, 83, 2
Yuthok the Elder, see Yuthok Yönten Gönpo 2, 42
Yuthok the Younger, see Yuthok Yönten Gönpo 2, 7, 45, 48
Yuthok Yönten Gönpo 45, 55

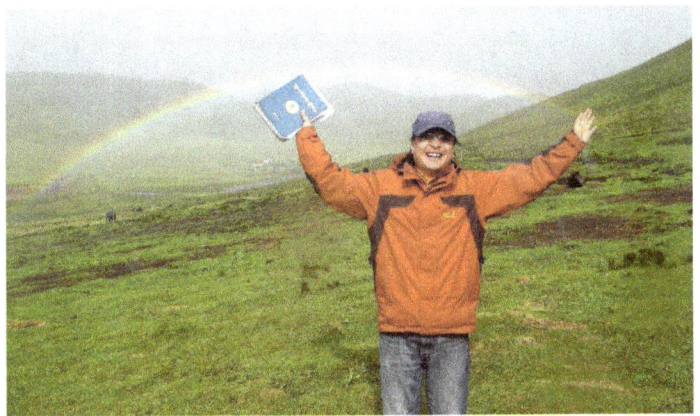

Dr. Nida Chenagtsang, a Tibetan doctor, Director of the International Academy for Traditional Tibetan Medicine (IATTM) is trained in modern and Traditional Tibetan Medicine, and seen his writings translated into nine languages.

He is dedicated to training students globally in a comprehensive four year Tibetan Medicine program, as well as in other modalities such as Ku Nye Massage, External Therapies, Mantra Healing, Nejang Healing Yoga, traveling tirelessly throughout Asia, Europe and the Americas to help set up over 25 International Academies for Traditional Tibetan Medicine (IATTM).

He has published many articles and books on ancient Tibetan Medicine, establishing important research areas and bringing back into current usage long forgotten traditional therapies. A founder of the Ngak Mang Institute, he has also helped preserve and disseminate the Ngakpa culture in modern Tibetan society today.

www.ingramcontent.com/pod-product-compliance
Lightning Source LLC
LaVergne TN
LVHW021119080426
835510LV00012B/1763